Nutritional support for adults and children

A handbook for hospital practice

Edited by

Tim Bowling

Consultant in Clinical Nutrition and Gastroenterology
Queen's Medical Centre
Nottingham

Radcliffe Medical Press

Radcliffe Medical Press Ltd
18 Marcham Road
Abingdon
Oxon OX14 1AA
United Kingdom

www.radcliffe-oxford.com
The Radcliffe Medical Press electronic catalogue and online ordering facility.
Direct sales to anywhere in the world.

British Library Cataloguing in Publication Data

A catalogue record for this book is available from the British Library.

ISBN 1 85775 831 5

Typeset by Aarontype Ltd, Easton, Bristol
Printed and bound by TJ International Ltd, Padstow, Cornwall

Contents

Foreword

Dr Bowling and his team are to be congratulated on responding so precisely to the brief provided for them by the Council of the British Association for Parenteral and Enteral Nutrition (BAPEN). BAPEN has long recognised that there is a dearth of knowledge about clinical nutrition and nutritional support in hospital settings, and has wished to address this in a practical and non-threatening fashion. There are of course many worthy tomes and specialty-specific reference manuals, but in my opinion none of these so effectively bridges the gaps between dietitian, doctor, nurse and pharmacist, nor provides such a commendably brief *vade mecum* for day-to-day clinical practice. Dr Bowling finds it necessary to justify a very basic approach and I agree with his logic, but in fact there is much in this small book to educate even the more experienced practitioner. This becomes especially true when we consider the advice given on conditions that may only occasionally be encountered in a given unit, and most obviously so for the adult specialist called upon to give advice in a difficult paediatric case. I recommend the book highly and feel confident that well-thumbed and battered copies will soon be found on wards everywhere.

Alastair Forbes
Chairman of BAPEN

Foreword

Good nutrition is essential for wellbeing and recovery from illness or injury. Technical advances mean that more patients than ever before are able to receive nutritional support. Unfortunately practical teaching and information in its use are often still sparse. For those not specialising in the field of clinical nutrition the array of tubes, feeds, routes etc that can provide nutrition may often seem bewildering. This book should help those non-specialists to make appropriate choices regarding nutritional care for their patients, including identifying those at risk, and choosing the most suitable route, access device and feed. Advice regarding ongoing assessment and prevention, detection and treatment of some complications of therapy is also given.

Although based on theoretical concepts the emphasis of the book is on practical day-to-day issues. It should prove to be a valuable resource for all professions, in many areas of practice.

Lynne Colagiovanni
Chairman, National Nurses Nutrition Group

Foreword

Nutritional problems can affect most parts of the body, and at times of illness providing appropriate nutritional care for patients is paramount to recovery. All healthcare professionals working with patients in hospitals should be aware of the importance of addressing the nutritional aspects of care when considering the clinical management of the patient. All too often this important area of care is neglected but having rapid access to key nutritional facts and information can help practitioners to address this issue.

The authors are to be congratulated on compiling this much needed comprehensive clinical nutrition guide for busy healthcare professionals working at ward level. It covers all aspects of nutritional care in a logical and systematic way and will aid clinicians in making reasoned judgements about the initial nutritional care that their patients require.

This succinct guide will be a valuable resource for clinicians of all grades (however experienced) who need rapid access to up-to-date facts on the nutritional considerations that are important for a wide range of clinical conditions.

This guide is written principally for ward doctors and nurses but dietitians will also find it an extremely useful addition to the reference materials and tools that they use on a daily basis in their everyday work.

Vera Todorovic
The Parenteral and Enteral Nutrition Group of the
British Dietetic Association

Foreword

The provision of adequate nutrition is now an accepted aspect of every patient's care for a multitude of professional groups. As more aggressive approaches are used for artificial nutritional support so the need for practical advice increases and this handbook certainly bridges the gap.

The multidisciplinary input into this book reflects what is necessary to optimise nutritional support and provides guidance on the practical application of the available evidence. We congratulate the authors on their ability to summarise a vast amount of information into such a useful handbook format.

Pharmacists are becoming increasingly involved in nutritional aspects of patient therapy. However, formal teaching on this subject is still limited. This handbook will be an invaluable resource, as it provides a concise, practical guide covering all aspects of clinical nutrition, both for adult and paediatric patients. It allows junior staff from all professions to understand the subject and make a positive impact on patient care.

Rebecca White, Vicky Bradnam
British Pharmaceutical Nutrition Group

Preface

Effective management of undernutrition requires an adequate knowledge base on the part of healthcare professionals. For many ward-based doctors and nurses this is inadequate, as nutrition has until recently been insufficiently addressed in training curricula. Consequently nutritional care in many UK and European hospitals is sub-optimal.

Although there is a great deal of literature and publications to assist the interested and informed, there is very little to aid the busy and less well informed.

This book has been commissioned by BAPEN to serve as a basic-level text aimed specifically at ward-based clinical and nursing staff at all levels of seniority. It is designed to be succinct and clear and to facilitate best practice.

It has been written by a multidisciplinary group of authors and we hope that it will be a useful and informative publication.

Dr Tim Bowling
(on behalf of the writing group)
2003

List of contributors

Vicky Blackshaw BSc, SRD, Senior Dietitian, University Hospital of North Staffordshire NHS Trust, Stoke-on-Trent.

Tim Bowling MD FRCP, Consultant in Clinical Nutrition and Gastroenterology, Queen's Medical Centre, University Hospital NHS Trust, Nottingham.

Claire Brady RGN, ENB100, BSc, MSc, Nutrition Nurse Specialist, Royal Free Hospital NHS Trust, London.

Katie Durman BSc, SRD, Chief Dietitian, Barts and The London NHS Trust, London.

Carole Glencorse BSc, SRD, DipADP, Nutritional Services Manager, Abbott Laboratories Ltd, Maidenhead.

Lindsay Harper BSc(Hons), DipClin, MRPharmS, Clinical Pharmacist for Intestinal Failure, Hope Hospital, Manchester.

Chris Holden RGN, RSCN, MSc, Paediatric Nutrition Nurse Specialist, Princess Diana Children's Hospital, Birmingham.

Sara McDowell BSc, SRD, DipADP, Senior Specialist Paediatric Dietitian, Leicester Royal Infirmary, Leicester.

John Puntis BM(Hons), DM, FRCP, FRCPCH, Senior Lecturer in Paediatrics and Child Health, University of Leeds, and Consultant Paediatric Gastroenterologist, The General Infirmary at Leeds, Leeds.

Lyndsay Raine BSc, MRPharmS, Principal Pharmacist, Royal Manchester Children's Hospital, Manchester.

Alastair Windsor MD, FRCS, FRCS(Ed), Consultant Surgeon, St Mark's Hospital, Harrow.

Acknowledgements

Thanks are due to the Child Growth Foundation for their permission to reproduce the BMI Chart in Chapter 3 and the boys and girls height and weight charts in Chapter 8.

PART 1

Introduction to undernutrition

CHAPTER 1

Introduction

Malnutrition is a problem endemic in all countries, and encompasses both under- and overnutrition. This book concerns itself exclusively with undernutrition.

At least 20–30% of patients in European hospitals are undernourished, or at risk of becoming so as a result of their illness. Undernutrition increases complications and costs of care, and is therefore a very significant pressure on healthcare delivery.

To minimise the impact of undernutrition in hospitalised patients, effective and appropriate management must be achieved. Traditionally, certainly in the UK, nutrition has been poorly taught to nurses and at both undergraduate and postgraduate levels to doctors. As a result there is a great deal of ignorance and poor practice at all levels of seniority. Better education in this field is beginning to bear fruit, but there is still a long way to go.

With regards to the practice of nutritional support, multidisciplinary nutrition teams are an ideal means of delivering and leading best practice. However, despite a growing recognition of their benefits to patient care, both in the literature and also by national organisations, less than 50% of UK hospitals and even fewer in many European countries have them. Even where they do exist they are often poorly resourced and can usually only help with a relatively small proportion of patients, who will invariably be at the 'high tech' end of the spectrum, e.g. those on intravenous (IV) feeding. Dietitians are another key group, but their numbers are also limited and they cannot see everyone who needs nutritional input. Therefore, the majority of patients rely on ward-based doctors and nurses in all disciplines to look out for, identify and manage undernutrition, and to refer on to more experienced professionals, i.e. dietitians and nutrition teams, those that require particular help.

The abilities and experience of ward-based staff in recognising and managing nutrition-related illness are very poor. This book is therefore aimed specifically at clinicians (from medical student to consultant) and ward nurses (from student to ward sister). We make no apology for pitching it at a very basic level, because it is core knowledge that is lacking and, without this, best practice is not going to be achievable. For the interested reader, there are specific references in the further reading list at the end of each section, and some more generic nutrition references at the end of this chapter.

The book is broadly split into two parts, one dealing with adult-based practice and the other with paediatrics. The same topics are covered. Overall, the intention is to present a brief and succinct but up-to-date guide which will both inform and enable the target readership to improve and optimise their knowledge and practice of nutritional support in the hospital setting.

We have attempted to base any practice recommendations on the highest level of authority that is available. Sometimes this is consensus within and between national organisations. Often, though, such consensus does not exist, for example with peri-operative nutritional support, and then recommendations can only be on the basis of expert opinion. More explicit details for particular situations can be found in the references at the end of each section.

Throughout the book there are examples of practical management of procedures and various clinical situations. In many hospitals there may be local protocols/guidelines. Where these exist they should be referred to.

Further reading

- Lennard-Jones JE (ed) (1992) *A Positive Approach to Nutrition as Treatment. Report of a working party*. King's Fund, London.
- Mann J and Truswell AS (eds) (2002) *Essentials of Human Nutrition*. Oxford University Press, Oxford.
- Payne-James JJ, Grimble GK and Silk DBA (eds) (2001) *Artificial Nutritional Support in Clinical Practice*. Greenwich Medical Media, London.
- Royal College of Physicians (2002) *Nutrition and Patients: a doctor's responsibility. Report of a working party of the Royal College of Physicians*. Royal College of Physicians, London.
- Stratton RJ, Green CJ and Elia M (2003) *Disease-related Malnutrition: an evidence-based approach to treatment*. CABI Publishing, Wallingford.
- Todorovic V and Micklewright A (eds) (2000) *Pocket Guide to Clinical Nutrition*. British Dietetic Association, London.

BAPEN, Maidenhead, publications

- Allison SP (ed) (1999) *Hospital Food as Treatment*.
- BAPEN working party (2003) *Drug Administration* via *Enteral Feeding Tubes*.
- Lennard-Jones JE (ed) (1998) *Ethical and Legal Aspects of Clinical Hydration and Nutritional Support*.
- McAtear C (ed) (1999) *Current Perspectives on Enteral Nutrition in Adults*.
- Milla PJ (ed) (2000) *Current Perspectives on Paediatric Parenteral Nutrition*.
- Pennington CJ (ed) (1996) *Current Perspectives on Parenteral Nutrition in Adults*.
- Silk DBA (ed) (1994) *Organisation of Nutritional Support in Hospitals*.
- Sizer T (ed) (1996) *Standards and Guidelines for Nutritional Support*.

CHAPTER 2

Undernutrition

Incidence

Undernutrition in hospitals has been a common problem for some time. It usually results from a deficit between intake and requirements over a period of time. The primary feature is a loss of body weight, due to depletion of body fat and muscle stores (protein–energy malnutrition). This contributes to patient morbidity and mortality.

A number of studies has consistently indicated that 20–40% of hospitalised patients are undernourished. This figure is probably an underestimate of true prevalence, as it does not include patients who were too ill on admission to be assessed.

Once in hospital undernutrition is likely to get worse, with approximately two-thirds losing weight while an in-patient.

Consequences of nutritional deficiencies

- Impaired immune function and risk of infection/sepsis.
- Delayed wound healing, increased risk of post-operative complications.
- Increased risk of pressure ulcers.
- Muscle wasting and weakness which in turn affects:
  - respiratory function → chest infections
  - cardiac function → heart failure
  - mobility → ↑ risk of deep vein thrombosis/pulmonary embolus and pressure ulcers
  - apathy, depression, self-neglect
  - general weakness which impairs physical ability to eat.

Overall undernutrition leads to longer length of stay in hospital and increased costs of care.

Risk factors for undernutrition

Risk factors, which may contribute to the development of undernutrition, can be split into three categories (*see* Box 2.1).

1 Decreased dietary intake.
2 Increased nutritional requirements.
3 Impaired absorption or utilisation of nutrients.

Box 2.1 Risk factors for undernutrition

1 *Factors which may decrease dietary intake.*
   • Difficulties with preparation/shopping/eating food due to illness or limited mobility.
   • Reduced appetite resulting from illness/anxiety/depression.
   • Symptoms associated with disease or treatments, e.g. nausea, vomiting, sore mouth or diarrhoea.
   • Lack of interest in food due to bereavement, isolation or mental illness.
   • Inadequate, unappetising foods.
   • Repeated fasting for treatments or procedures.
   • Swallowing/chewing difficulties, e.g. due to poor fitting dentures.
   • Difficulty self-feeding.
   • Semi-consciousness.
2 *Increased nutritional requirements.*
   • During metabolic stress nutritional requirements and utilisation of nutrients are increased.
   • Wound/fistula losses.
3 *Impaired ability to absorb or utilise nutrients.*
   • Due to disease or treatment, e.g. coeliac disease, malabsorption, intestinal resection.
   • Enzyme deficiencies.
   • Intraluminal factors, e.g. high/low pH.
   • Motility abnormalities.
   • Infection, e.g. parasites, gastroenteritis.

Further reading

• Bettany G and Powell-Tuck J (1995) Malnutrition: incidence, diagnosis, causes, effects and indications for nutritional support. *Eur J Gastroent Hepatol.* **7**: 494–500.
• Corish CA and Kennedy NP (2000) Protein–energy undernutrition in hospital in-patients. *Br J Nutr.* **83**: 575–91.
• Edington J, Boorman J, Durrant E *et al.* (2000) Prevalence of malnutrition on admission to four hospitals in England. *Clin Nutr.* **19**: 191–5.
• McWhirter JP and Pennington CR (1994) Incidence and recognition of malnutrition in hospital. *BMJ.* **308**: 945–58.
• Vetta A, Ronzoni S, Taglieri G *et al.* (1999) The impact of malnutrition on the quality of life in the elderly. *Clin Nutr.* **18**: 259–67.

PART 2

Adults

CHAPTER 3

Nutritional assessment

Introduction

Nutritional assessment is used to:

- determine nutritional status and identify patients likely to benefit from nutritional support
- determine goals of nutritional support
- act as a baseline against which nutritional management can be monitored.

Although there is no single way of defining undernutrition the factors detailed below are useful in identifying it.

If undernutrition is identified, or a patient is assessed to be at risk of becoming undernourished, it is essential that appropriate action is taken. Hospitals should have protocols in place to identify such patients and direct appropriate ongoing nutritional management, which will invariably involve dietitians ± nutrition teams.

Method of assessment
Weight loss

In the absence of oedema or ascites body weight is a useful measurement of nutritional status. If oedema or ascites is present, it is possible to determine dry weight using the guide below (*see* Table 3.1).

Rapid alteration in weight within days rather than weeks is most likely to be fluid.

$$\text{Percentage weight loss} = \frac{(\text{usual weight kg} - \text{actual weight kg})}{\text{usual weight kg}} \times 100$$

See Table 3.2 for the significance of weight loss as a percentage of pre-illness weight.

Table 3.1 Guidelines for estimating fluid weight in patients with ascites and oedema

	Oedema	Ascites
Minimal	1.0 kg	2.2 kg
Moderate	5.0 kg	6.0 kg
Severe	10.0 kg	14.0 kg

Table 3.2   The significance of weight loss as a percentage of pre-illness weight

% Weight change (over 3–6 months)	Interpretation
<5	Within normal intra-individual variation
5–10	More than normal intra-individual variation – early indicator of increased risk of undernutrition
>10	Clinically significant, requires nutritional support

Body mass index

- Body mass index (BMI) – *see* Figure 3.1 – gives a rapid interpretation of chronic protein–energy status based on the individual's height and weight.
- Where height and/or weight are not available, self-reported height or weight can be used if these are reasonable or realistic. If these measures are unobtainable, subjective criteria should be used to form an overall clinical impression of nutritional risk, e.g. are clothing or rings loose?
- BMI can be calculated as follows:

$$\text{BMI} = \frac{\text{weight kg}}{(\text{height m})^2}$$

BMI may be interpreted as follows:

- $<18.5 \, \text{kg/m}^2$ underweight, chronic undernutrition probable
- $18.5–20 \, \text{kg/m}^2$ underweight, chronic undernutrition possible
- $20–25 \, \text{kg/m}^2$ desirable weight, chronic malnutrition unlikely
- $25–30 \, \text{kg/m}^2$ overweight, increased risk of complications associated with chronic overnutrition
- $>30 \, \text{kg/m}^2$ obese, moderate ($30–35 \, \text{kg/m}^2$), high ($35–40 \, \text{kg/m}^2$) and very high risk ($>40 \, \text{kg/m}^2$) of obesity-related complications.

It should be appreciated that BMI measurements in older people are not as accurate as they do not take into account loss of height with age or loss of muscle mass. Nevertheless they are still widely used in the elderly. There are alternative methods of assessing nutritional status in the elderly, such as demispan (sternal notch to web of ring and middle fingers), but these are not utilised widely and further detail has therefore not been included here.

Anthropometry

Anthropometry measures lean body mass and body fat stores. These measurements are useful in assessing body composition in patients with ascites or oedema, or in those who cannot be weighed. As changes in body composition take place

Body Mass Index Chart

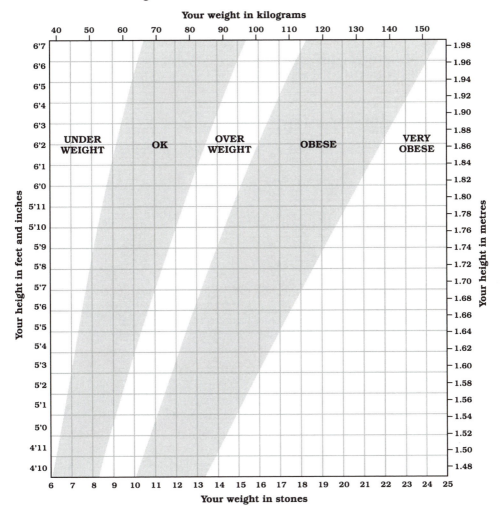

Figure 3.1 BMI chart.

slowly, then these techniques tend only to be used with patients on long-term nutritional support, or for research purposes. All measurements should be taken by appropriately trained personnel, e.g. dietitians.

Anthropometric measurements commonly used include:

- mid arm circumference (MAC): simple estimate of muscle mass
- triceps skinfold thickness (TSF): measure of fat stores
- mid arm muscle circumference (MAMC): can be calculated using the following formula and provides an indication of skeletal muscle mass:

$$\text{MAMC (cm)} = \text{MAC (cm)} - 3.14 \times \text{TSF (cm)}.$$

Grip strength can be measured using a hand-grip dynamometer and is a functional measure of muscle function. This technique may be used with patients receiving long-term nutritional support but is limited by the fact that the technique relies on patient motivation and compliance.

Bio-impedance analysis may be used to assess body composition. It relies on a steady hydration status, which may make it invalid in certain clinical states. This is very much a research tool.

Dietary considerations

Consider whether a patient is meeting their requirements by looking at:

- current food/fluid intake *versus* requirements
- changes in appetite
- presence of factors which may affect oral intake (*see* Box 2.1).

Clinical considerations

The following factors may contribute to nutrient deficiencies.

- Increased requirements, e.g. fever, metabolic stress.
- Increased nutrient losses, e.g. vomiting, diarrhoea, renal excretion, haemorrhage and wound/fistula losses.
- Impaired digestion/absorption, e.g. pancreatitis, coeliac disease.

Consider:

- physical appearance, e.g. emaciation, hair loss, or loose clothing, rings or dentures, which are indicative of weight loss
- presence of peripheral oedema, ascites, dry non-elastic skin.

Biochemical measurements

Albumin
Albumin is a poor marker of nutritional status. Protein–energy malnutrition causes a decrease in albumin synthesis but, as it has a very long half life of 21 days, changes due to poor nutrition are slow. Falls in serum albumin are more likely to occur secondary to disease state or changes in hydration, such as:

- catabolic/septic/inflammatory states
- as a result of dilution from IV fluids
- increased excretion, e.g. nephrotic syndrome, malabsorption or inflammatory conditions of the intestine ($\uparrow$ gut losses)
- impaired hepatic synthesis.

The first two points listed above are the most common explanations of hypo-albuminaemia, especially when levels have dropped over a matter of days; i.e. when an albumin is 20 g/l 4 days post-operatively when it was 40 g/l pre-operatively, the explanation is due to a combination of fluid dilution and the expected catabolic state of the post-operative patient.

*Low albumin levels taken in isolation are **not** a marker of malnutrition.*

Transferrin
Transferrin has a half life of 8–10 days. However, its main function is to bind and transport iron. Therefore it is affected by iron status and the acute phase response.

Prealbumin
Prealbumin is more sensitive to protein depletion (with a half life of 2–3 days) but is also extremely sensitive to changes in metabolic stress and disease.

Retinol-binding protein
Retinol-binding protein has a short half life of 12 hours and its indications are similar to that of prealbumin. However, it is technically very difficult to measure and not widely available.

Nutritional screening

Nutritional screening is a way of identifying patients who are undernourished or at risk of becoming undernourished. The hospital admission process should include nutritional screening for all patients by nursing or medical staff or healthcare assistants. Screening should be repeated at weekly intervals for the hospitalised patient unless a patient is identified as being at high risk, in which case he/she should be referred to a dietitian for further assessment.

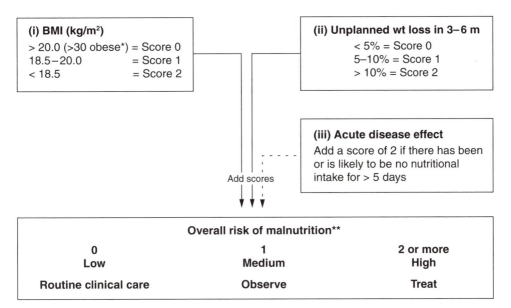

*Follow local policy.   **See Box 3.1.

Figure 3.2 'Malnutrition Universal Screening Tool' ('MUST') for adults.

Box 3.1   'Malnutrition Universal Screening Tool' ('MUST') for adults

- *If height, weight or weight loss cannot be established*:
  - use documented or recalled values (if realistic)
  - when measured or recalled height cannot be obtained, use an alternative measure (e.g. ulna length, knee height). Otherwise, obtain an overall impression of whether the patient is at risk of malnutrition (no/low risk [note obesity] *versus* increased risk) using the following as a guide:
    - (i) *BMI*. Clinical impression (very thin/thin, acceptable, overweight/obese*) and mid upper arm circumference <23.5 cm (>32 cm for obese*)
    - (ii) *weight change*. Clothes and/or jewellery have become loose fitting (weight loss) or too tight (weight gain); history of changes in food intake, appetite or dysphagia over 3–6 months and underlying disease or psychosocial/physical disabilities likely to cause weight change
    - (iii) *acute disease*. No nutritional intake for >5 days.
- *Low risk – routine clinical care. Repeat screening.*
  - Hospital – every week.
  - Care homes – every month.
  - Community – every year for special groups, e.g. those >75 years of age.
  - *Obese – follow local policy.
- *Medium risk – observe.*
  - Hospital – document dietary and fluid intake for 3 days.
  - Care homes (as for hospital).
  - Community – repeat screening, e.g. from <1 month to >6 months (with dietary advice if necessary).
- *High risk – treat.*
  - Hospital – refer to dietitian or implement local policies. Consider dietary fortification and supplements.
  - Care homes (as for hospital).
  - Community (as for hospital).

There are many variations of nutritional screening tools used. Figure 3.2 and Box 3.1 illustrate the 'Malnutrition Universal Screening Tool' ('MUST') recently devised and validated by BAPEN. 'MUST' needs to be accompanied by a care plan agreed locally.

Further reading

- Arrowsmith H (1999) A critical evaluation of the use of nutrition screening tools by nurses. *Br J Nurs*. **8**: 1483–90.
- Beck A and Ovesen L (1998) At which body mass index and degree of weight loss should hospitalized elderly patients be considered at nutritional risk? *Clin Nutr*. **17**: 195–8.

- Carney DE and Meguid MM (2002) Current concepts in nutritional assessment. *Arch Surg.* **137**: 42–5.
- Guigoz Y, Lauque S and Vellas BJ (2002) Identifying the elderly at risk for malnutrition. The Mini Nutritional Assessment. *Clin Geriatr Med.* **8**: 737–57.
- Jeejeebhoy KN (2000) Nutritional assessment. *Nutrition.* **16**: 585–90.
- McClave SA, McClain CJ and Snider HL (2001) Should indirect calorimetry be used as part of nutritional assessment? *J Clin Gastroenterol.* **33**: 14–19.
- Perissinotto E, Pisent C, Sergi G *et al.* (2002) Anthropometric measurements in the elderly: age and gender differences. *Br J Nutr.* **87**: 177–86.
- Ravasco P, Camilo ME, Gouveia-Oliveira A *et al.* (2002) A critical approach to nutritional assessment in critically ill patients. *Clin Nutr.* **21**: 73–7.
- Selberg O and Sel S (2001) The adjunctive value of routine biochemistry in nutritional assessment of hospitalized patients. *Clin Nutr.* **20**: 477–85.

CHAPTER 4

Nutritional requirements

Introduction

Undernutrition may result from a deficiency of macronutrients or micronutrients. It is therefore important to consider nutrient needs (*see* Box 4.1).

Box 4.1   Nutrients required

- Macronutrients.
  - Protein.
  - Fat.
  - Carbohydrate.
- Micronutrients.
  - Vitamins.
  - Trace elements.
- (Water + electrolytes.)

Energy

Energy expenditure consists of three components.

1 Resting energy expenditure (REE).
2 Metabolic requirements in health and disease.
3 Thermic effects of food, i.e. the energy required to utilise macronutrients.

In the hospitalised patient eating relatively little, the thermic effects of food are modest, and hence the main components of energy expenditure are REE and metabolic requirements.

Energy supply is mostly derived from metabolism of carbohydrate, fat and protein, and is measured in kcal.

Supplying inadequate energy results in tissue breakdown; supplying too much leads to increased storage as glycogen or fat. Neither of these is desirable, either in health or disease. The aim therefore is energy balance, which means that intake and expenditure are in equilibrium. This implies that calculation of energy requirements is of fundamental importance. Calculation of energy requirements is best done by calorimetry, but the cost of equipment and time involved make its use impractical. Three more practical methods are described below, two of which entail calculations of REE with added factors to take into account the clinical situation of the patient.

'Rule of thumb'

This is a more crude method of estimating requirements than the formulae described below, but for busy ward staff it is a useful guide.

- Energy requirements:
  - 25–35 kcal/kg/day
  - 25 kcal/kg/day: bedbound, but not catabolic, i.e. apyrexial, non-surgical
  - 30 kcal/kg/day: pyrexial or post-operative
  - 35 kcal/kg/day: pyrexial and post-operative, multiple trauma.
- If weight gain is required add at least 200 kcal to total daily requirements.
- If weight loss is required subtract at least 200 kcal from total daily requirements.

The Harris Benedict equation

The Harris Benedict equation estimates basal energy expenditure (BEE), i.e. the energy expended by a fasting person at rest in a thermoneutral environment. Estimation of BEE is calculated as follows.

Males   (kcal/24 hours) = $66.5 + (13.8\,W) + (5\,H) - (6.8\,A)$

Females   (kcal/24 hours) = $655 + (9.6\,W) + (1.8\,H) - (4.7\,A)$

Where W = weight in kg; H = height in metres, A = age in years

Stress factors. (*See* Table 4.1 for multiples which need to be added to convert BEE into REE.)

Table 4.1   Multiples to be added to convert BEE into REE

Stress factor	*Multiple*
Post-operative (no complications)	1.0
Peritonitis/sepsis	1.1–1.3
Severe infection/multiple trauma	1.2–1.4
Burns	1.2–2.0

The Schofield equation

This is perhaps the most commonly used equation in the UK employed to predict basal metabolic rate (BMR), and it is used in conjunction with the Elia nomogram to give an estimation of energy requirements including stress factors. Once BMR has been estimated (*see* Table 4.2), adjust for stress using the nomogram (*see* Figure 4.1), and add a factor for activity and dietary induced thermogenesis (*see* Table 4.3).

Table 4.2 Equations for estimating BMR (Schofield)

Females kcal/day	Males kcal/day
15–18 years 13.3 W + 690	15–18 years 17.6 W + 656
18–30 years 14.8 W + 485	18–30 years 15.0 W + 690
30–60 years 8.1 W + 842	30–60 years 11.4 W + 870
Over 60 years 9.0 W + 656	Over 60 years 11.7 W + 585

W = Weight in kg.

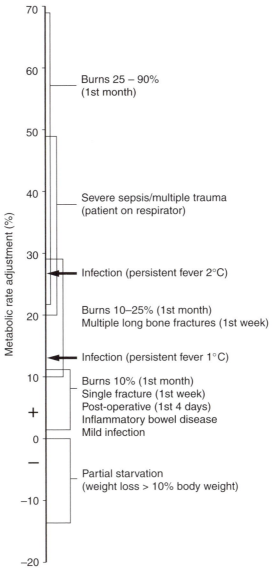

Figure 4.1 Method for estimating the approximate energy and nutrition requirements in adult patients receiving artificial nutritional support. Reproduced from Elia M (1990) Artificial nutritional support. *Medicine*. **82**. By kind permission of the Medicine Publishing Group.

Table 4.3 Activity factor for the Schofield equation

Bedbound immobile	+ 10%
Bedbound mobile/sitting	+ 15–20%
Mobile on ward	+ 25%

Protein

Protein provides amino acids essential for growth and continuous replacement of body tissues and enzymes.

When amino acids are broken down, nitrogen is released and excreted, primarily in the form of urea. If nitrogen intake equals excretion an individual is in nitrogen balance. Where more nitrogen is excreted this is a negative nitrogen balance, and occurs in catabolic processes, such as the post-operative or critically ill patient. A positive nitrogen balance is retaining more nitrogen than excreting, and indicates new tissue synthesis. This is essential in growing children, pregnancy and recovery from illness.

- 1 g of protein yields 4 kcal energy.
- Total dietary energy from protein should be 15–20%.
- Reference nutrient intake for protein in a healthy adult is 0.75 g/kg body weight/day.
- Protein contains 16% nitrogen. To convert grams of nitrogen to grams of protein multiply the nitrogen value by 6.25.
- In obese people, using actual body weight to calculate protein requirements would overestimate needs. It is therefore recommended that, for people with a BMI greater than 30 kg/m^2, either 75% of protein requirements determined from actual body weight or 130% of ideal body weight should be used.
- Metabolic stress increases protein requirements, and it is often difficult to achieve positive nitrogen balance in metabolically stressed patients, e.g. post-operatively.
- Calculation of nitrogen losses requires equipment not widely available. However, on occasions it is important to assess this, especially in the patient on longer-term nutritional support, when it is necessary to calculate more accurately protein requirements. A simpler measure of nitrogen losses can be calculated by the following formula:

$$\text{Nitrogen loss} = \text{urinary 24 hour urea excretion (mmol)} \times 0.028 + 2$$

The + 2 in the above formula represents an approximation of non-urinary urea losses, e.g. faeces, skin, wound. This formula is not that accurate, but on the whole it is good enough for the purposes of practical nutritional management.
- Traditionally the energy content of parenteral nutrition (PN) solutions is expressed as non-protein energy, i.e. the calories supplied by fat and carbohydrate only. This is because it is assumed that the protein source is protected from utilisation for energy if carbohydrate and fat provision is adequate. When

Table 4.4   Guide for estimating requirements

Metabolic state	Nitrogen g/kg/day	Protein g/kg/day
'Normal', i.e. no catabolic illness	0.13–0.16	0.8–1.0
Post-operative (no complications)	0.16–0.19	1.0–1.2
Post-operative + septic complications	0.19–0.22	1.2–1.4
Severe sepsis/multiple organ failure/burns	0.22–0.32	1.4–2.0

assessing nutritional requirements for patients receiving PN, you should check with the pharmacist to see whether bags are formulated based on total energy or non-protein energy. For patients on an oral diet or enteral feeding it can be assumed that energy is expressed as total calories, i.e. includes calories from protein.

- *See* Table 4.4 for a guide on estimating requirements.

Carbohydrates

Carbohydrate is rapidly broken down to glucose and is the most readily available source of energy to the body.

- 1 g carbohydrate yields 3.75 kcal energy.
- Glucose requirements for both healthy and 'stable' sick individuals are similar and can be set at 4–5 g/kg/day, and constitute on average 50% of total dietary energy.
- Glucose comes either from exogenous carbohydrate (i.e. oral or IV) or from internal metabolic processes. It is stored as glycogen in the liver and skeletal muscles, but these reserves are usually exhausted after 24–36 hours of starvation. Thereafter glucose comes from amino acids (gluconeogenesis), fat (lipolysis) and lactate (product of anaerobic energy utilisation).
- Excess glucose is stored either as glycogen or converted into fatty acids and stored as triglycerides in the liver and adipose tissue.
- The body has an oxidative capacity, i.e. a limit beyond which the body is unable to utilise glucose. Carbohydrate given to excess cannot be oxidised and can therefore be detrimental. This will lead to hepatic accumulation of both glycogen and fat and consequent cholestasis and organ dysfunction.
- When cells 'use' glucose as a source of energy – glucose oxidation – carbon dioxide is released. This CO_2 then has to be excreted mainly from the lungs. More CO_2 is produced from glucose oxidation than from either fat or protein. Therefore the higher the proportion of energy supplied by carbohydrate the greater the CO_2 production. This can have implications for patients with respiratory disease or on ventilators. If this may be of clinical relevance, low carbohydrate enteral feeds can be used.

Table 4.5   Adult requirements for water and electrolytes

	Baseline requirement		Other considerations
	Oral	IV	
Water			
Maintenance	18–60 yrs 35 ml/kg body weight 60 yrs 30 ml/kg body weight	As oral	Additional bicarbonate may be required in individuals with biliary, pancreatic, small bowel and diarrhoeal fluid loss. This needs to be given separately and not as a component of the enteral or parenteral feeds
Replacement of losses: Fever	Add 2–2.5 ml/kg/day for each °C rise in body temp above 37°C		
Body fluids	Assess on individual basis		
Electrolytes			
Sodium	60–100 mmol/day (1.0 mmol/kg)	1–1.5 mmol/kg/24 hr (1 litre of 0.9% normal saline contains 150 mmol NaCl)	Add 1.5 mmol sodium to each 10 ml additional fluid required as calculated above. Unless clinically indicated enteral and parenteral feeds should contain a minimum of 50 mmol sodium/day
Potassium	50–100 mmol/day (1.0 mmol/kg)	1–1.5 mmol/kg/24 hr Need more if serum potassium levels <3.5 mmol or refeeding severely malnourished patients	Additional potassium may be required if serum potassium is low

Calcium	20 mmol/day (0.2 mmol/kg)	0.1–0.15 mmol/kg/24 hr	Calcium correction – a low plasma calcium level may be due to a decrease in the transport protein albumin as approximately 50% of calcium is protein bound. To correct total calcium for changes in albumin: corrected calcium = measured calcium (mmol) + (40 – serum albumin g/l)/40
Magnesium	12–14 mmol/day (0.2 mmol/kg)	0.1–0.2 mmol/kg/24 hr	May require extra with large gastrointestinal losses or refeeding malnourished patients
Phosphate	25 mmol/day (0.3 mmol/kg)	0.5–0.7 mmol/kg/24 hr or 10 mmol/1000 kcal feed	Do not exceed 50 mmol phosphate/day in enteral or parenteral feed. Correct hypophosphataemia before initiating enteral nutrition or PN
Chloride	60–100 mmol/day (1.0 mmol/kg)	1–1.5 mmol/kg/24 hr	

Table 4.6   Suggested vitamin, mineral and trace element requirements for adults

Element	Oral/enteral requirements (recommended daily amount)	IV requirements (recommended daily amount)	Function	Deficiency	Food sources
Electrolytes					
Calcium	See Table 4.5	See Table 4.5	Forms teeth and bones, muscle contraction	Muscle aches, pain, twitching, spasm, cramps, tetany, loose teeth/gum infection	Milk and dairy products, dark green vegetables, pulses, fish (with bones)
Phosphate	See Table 4.5	See Table 4.5	Bone development, release energy from food	Anorexia, lethargy, bone pain, calcification of soft tissue	Plant and animal foods
Magnesium	See Table 4.5	See Table 4.5	Bone development, muscle and nerve conduction, metabolism, DNA synthesis	Neuromuscular abnormalities, loss of appetite, nausea, vomiting, pre-menstrual syndrome, diarrhoea, numbness, tingling, dizziness, hypertension	Meat, fish, dairy products, green vegetables
Sodium	See Table 4.5	See Table 4.5	Maintenance of extracellular fluid volume	Muscle cramps, vertigo, nausea, apathy, reduced appetite	Processed foods, mineral water, table salt
Potassium	See Table 4.5	See Table 4.5	Acid base balance, nerve, muscle function	Muscle weakness/paralysis, cardiac arrest	Fruits, vegetables, dairy products, meat

Trace elements

Iron	8.7–10 mg	1.2 mg (20 μmol)	Blood formation	Fatigue, pallor, headache, dizziness, sore tongue/mouth, concave brittle nails	Red meat, offal, dark green vegetables
Zinc	9.5–15 mg	3.2–6.5 mg (50–100 μmol)	Metabolism, cell membranes	Poor growth, wound healing, eczema, psoriasis, acne, poor hair growth, increased risk of infection, delayed puberty, low sperm count, loss of smell, diarrhoea	Red meat, unrefined cereals
Copper	1.1–3.0 mg	0.3–1.3 mg (5–20 μmol)	Healthy skin, hair and red blood cells	Metabolic and muscle problems	Nuts, offal, oysters, vegetables
Iodine	140 μg	130 μg (1.0 μmol)	Metabolic rate maintenance, thyroid function	Lethargy, thyroid goitre, brittle course hair, weight gain, hypothyroidism	Seafood, dried seaweed, milk
Manganese	1–10 mg	0.2 mg (3–5 μmol)	Bone/tendon growth + synthesis of carbohydrate and proteins	Depression, weakness, leg cramps	Cereals, nuts, pulses, green vegetables
Fluoride	1.5–4.0 mg	0.1 mg (0–50 μmol)	Prevention of dental caries	Tooth decay, soft bones	Seafood, drinking water, tea
Chromium	50–200 μg	10–20 μg (0.2–0.4 μmol)	Energy metabolism, effective insulin action	Inability to metabolise glucose	Brewers yeast, wholegrain nuts, vegetables

Table 4.6 (continued)

Element	Oral/enteral requirements (recommended daily amount)	IV requirements (recommended daily amount)	Function	Deficiency	Food sources
Selenium	55–75 μg	30–60 μg (0.4–0.8 μmol)	Antioxidant	Muscle weakness, cardiomyopathy	Wholegrain cereals, meat, fish
Molybdenum	50–400 μg	19 μg (0.4 μmol)	Part of enzymes	Rare	Milk, legumes, cereals, kidney
Vitamins Vitamin A	700–1000 μg	1000 μg	Vision, bone/teeth formation, growth and tissue repair	Night blindness, keratomalacia, dry scaly skin, joint pain, fatigue, impaired growth and development in children	Dairy foods, fish liver oils, carrots, yellow and green vegetables
B₁ (thiamine)	0.9–1.2 mg	3 mg	Energy metabolism, appetite and nervous system function	Neurological disorders, confusion, cardiac irregularity, loss of appetite, fatigue, wet or dry beri-beri	Pork, poultry, fish, beans
B₂ (riboflavin)	1.3–1.6 mg	3.6 mg	Cell respiration, normal vision and skin	Lesions on mucocutaneous surfaces of mouth, skin rash, vascularisation of cornea	Meat, eggs, green vegetables, offal

			Function	Deficiency	Source
B_6 (pyridoxine)	1.4–2.0 mg	4.0 mg	Protein metabolism, sensory function	Glossitis, dermatitis, convulsions, muscle weakness, anaemia	Wholegrains, fish, meat, nuts, pulses
B_{12}	1.4–2.0 μg	5 μg	Cell synthesis, nerve myelination	Megaloblastic anaemia, fatigue, brain degeneration	Animal products
Niacin	15 mg	40 mg	Energy metabolism, healthy skin, nervous system and GI tract	Pellagra, fatigue, confusion	Meat, fish, dairy products, peanuts, yeast extract
Pantothenic acid	3–7 mg	10–20 mg	Release of energy from foods	Headache, dizziness, cramps, weakness, GI disturbance	Yeast, meats, wholegrains, vegetables
Biotin	10–200 μg	60 μg	Lipogenesis, gluconeogenesis, protein metabolism	Nausea, vomiting, depression, hair loss, dermatitis, mental and physical retardation in child development	Cereals, grains
Folate	200 μg	400 μg	Cell growth	GI disorders, macrocytic anaemia, neural tube defects in newborns	Liver, yeast extract, leafy green vegetables
Vitamin C (ascorbic acid)	40–60 mg	100 mg	Immunity, collagen formation, wound healing	Bleeding gums, scurvy, poor wound healing, bruising or haemorrhaging, fatigue, depression, muscle degeneration	Oranges, lemons, grapefruits, potatoes and tomatoes

Table 4.6 (continued)

Element	Oral/enteral requirements (recommended daily amount)	IV requirements (recommended daily amount)	Function	Deficiency	Food sources
Vitamin D	5 μg	5 μg	Development of bones and teeth, enhances absorption of calcium	Rickets in children, osteomalacia in adults, reduced teeth and bone development	Oily fish, egg yolks, offal, fortified margarine, sunlight on skin
Vitamin E	4–10 mg	10 mg	Antioxidant	Haemolytic anaemia, muscle wasting, reproductive failure, nerve damage	Wheatgerm, eggs, vegetable oils
Vitamin K	80 μg	150 μg	Blood clotting	Prolonged blood clotting time	Dairy foods, green vegetables, cereals

Fat

Fat is a more concentrated form of energy than carbohydrate or protein and also provides essential fatty acids.

- 1 g of fat yields 9 kcal energy.
- Dietary energy from fat should be around 35% of total energy intake. If too much fat is given (at the expense of carbohydrate) excessive lipolysis will occur leading to large amounts of circulating triglycerides, cholesterol and fatty acids, causing various metabolic problems. If too little fat is given (and therefore too much carbohydrate) there will be greater insulin release which will inhibit lipolysis, and lead to fat deposition. It is therefore important that the ratio of fat to carbohydrate calories does not stray out of the 40 : 60%–60 : 40% ratio.
- Lipid requirements in health and disease are approximately 1.0–1.5 g/kg/day.
- For critically ill patients lipid requirements are 0.8–1.0 g/kg/day. The lower amount is because of insulin resistance and hence less of an inhibiting effect on lipolysis (*see* p. 92).

Water and electrolytes

See Table 4.5 for adult requirements for water and electrolytes.

Vitamins, minerals and trace elements

Vitamins, minerals and trace elements (micronutrients) are essential for metabolism, tissue structure, enzyme systems, fluid balance and cellular function.

In order to provide effective nutritional support, nutritional requirements need to be known. Dietary reference values (DRVs) provide guidance on the nutritional requirements of the healthy population. These values are not, however, always appropriate to use with hospitalised patients, as they do not take into account factors such as infection, metabolic stress and pyrexia. Table 4.6 details all the micronutrients and relevant clinical facts. The amounts recommended for oral/enteral feeding are the DRVs; the amounts recommended for parenteral feeding are ranges, as it is still not clearly established for many of these nutrients exactly how much should be given.

Further reading

- Buttriss J (2000) Nutrient requirements and optimisation of intakes. *Br Med Bull.* **56**: 18–33.
- Department of Health (1991) *Report on Health and Social Subjects No 41. Dietary Reference Values for Food, Energy and Nutrients for the United Kingdom.* COMA HMSO, London.
- Elia M, Ritz P and Stubbs RJ (2000) Total energy expenditure in the elderly. *Eur J Clin Nutr.* **54** (Suppl 3): S92–103.
- Gibney ER (2000) Energy expenditure in disease: time to revisit? *Proc Nutr Soc.* **59**: 199–207.

- Kowanko I (2001) Energy and nutrient intake of patients in acute care. *Clin Nurs.* **10**: 51–7.
- Ritz P (2001) Factors affecting energy and macronutrient requirements in elderly people. *Public Health Nutr.* **4**: 561–8.
- Schofield WN (1985) Predicting basal metabolic rate, new standards and review of previous work. *Hum Nutr Clin Nutr.* **39** (Suppl 1): 5–41.
- Yates AA (2001) National nutrition and public health policies: issues related to bioavailability of nutrients when developing dietary reference intakes. *J Nutr.* **131** (Suppl 4): 1331S–4S.

CHAPTER 5

Methods of nutritional support

Introduction

Once a patient has been assessed and deemed in need of nutritional support, the next step is to determine the most appropriate method of feeding. The algorithm in Figure 5.1 illustrates the decision-making pathway, and demonstrates that simpler methods should always be considered first.

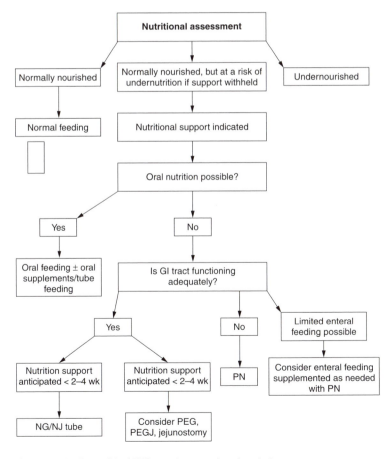

NG = nasogastric; NJ = nasojejunal; PEG = percutaneous endoscopic gastrostomy;
PEGJ = percutaneous endoscopic gastrojejunostomy; PN = parenteral nutrition.

Figure 5.1 Choices for nutritional support.

In this chapter are several examples of practical management. These should be read in conjunction with local policy/protocols where these exist.

Oral nutritional support
Food

Wherever possible the simplest approach should be used to improve nutritional intake and status. Food should always be considered first. Several recent initiatives and documents have made recommendations to improve the overall quality and access to food, to improve food provision and presentation at ward level and for food to be considered part of the patient's treatment: *Hospital Food as a Treatment* (BAPEN, 1999); *Essence of Care: patient-focused benchmarking* (DoH, 2001); and *Better Hospital Food: The NHS Plan* (DoH, 2000).

Strategies to increase nutritional intake from food in hospital include:

- providing high energy/high protein choices within the hospital menu and identifying these dishes on the menu so that patients can make informed choices
- offering a separate high protein/high energy menu for those identified as at risk of undernutrition
- fortifying ordinary foods to increase the protein and energy content, e.g. by adding cream, skimmed milk powder or cheese
- providing extra high protein/high energy snacks
- ensuring that meals are available for those who miss meal times due to procedures or theatre – missed meals make a big contribution to weight loss in hospital patients.

In order to target those at risk of undernutrition a screening tool can be used to identify patients at medium or high risk and help direct efforts to improve appropriate nutritional care and dietary intake. All hospitals should be using one such tool and all ward-based staff should familiarise themselves with it (*see* Chapter 3 for further details).

As well as providing appropriate food the environment should be conducive towards eating. Nicely presented food, clean tables, plates and cutlery, a day room for eating away from the bedside, and banning ward rounds at meal times are all examples of ways in which to improve the environment. Visitors can be both a help and a hindrance at meal times. This issue would need to be considered on an individual basis. Nurses, doctors and other staff have a crucial role in creating the right environment.

Further reading

- Allison SP (ed) (1999) *Hospital Food as a Treatment*. British Association for Parenteral and Enteral Nutrition, Maidenhead.
- American Dietetic Association (2001) Position of the American Dietetic Association: food fortification and dietary supplements. *J Am Diet Assoc*. **101**: 115–25.

- Department of Health (2000) *Better Hospital Food: The NHS Plan*. Department of Health, London.
- Department of Health (2001) *Essence of Care: patient-focused benchmarking for healthcare practitioners*. Department of Health, London.

Oral supplements

See Table 5.1 for the main types of oral nutritional supplements available, their properties and their indications for use.

Indications for the use of supplements
The use of oral supplements should be restricted to those who are unable to meet their nutritional requirements from ordinary food and drink. Attempts should be made to improve the nutritional content of the diet through high energy and high protein foods and drinks. If this approach fails or is unlikely to be sufficient, supplements should be tried. The use of oral nutritional supplements has been found to be effective in improving nutritional intake, nutritional status and, in some cases, outcome in a variety of clinical conditions. However, supplements are often used inappropriately and wasted, especially in the community. The involvement of a dietitian and regular review of the need for supplements can help to reduce wastage and costs.

Different types of supplements
There is a variety of nutritional supplements available, in liquid, semi-solid or powder form. Some are nutritionally complete, i.e. they provide all the main nutrients in a balanced way and can be taken as a supplement to the diet or as a sole source of nutrition. Others contain only some nutrients and are designed only to supplement the diet. When using supplements which are not nutritionally complete it is important to assess the nutrient content of the diet and ensure the supplement complements the current dietary intake. The patient's clinical condition may also affect the suitability of a particular supplement, e.g. those with renal failure may need a low volume, low electrolyte supplement. The dietitian is best placed to assess the nutritional content of the diet and advise on appropriate supplements.

Further reading
- American Dietetic Association (2001) Position of the American Dietetic Association: food fortification and dietary supplements. *J Am Diet Assoc*. **101**: 115–25.
- Green CJ (1999) Existence, causes and consequences of disease-related malnutrition in the hospital and community, and clinical and financial benefits of nutritional intervention. *Clin Nutr*. **18** (Suppl 2): 3–28.
- Potter J, Langhorne P and Roberts M (1998) Routine protein energy supplementation in adults: systematic review. *BMJ*. **317**: 495–501.
- Stratton RJ and Elia M (1999) A critical systematic analysis of the use of nutritional supplements in the community. *Clin Nutr*. **18** (Suppl 2): 29–84.

Table 5.1 The main types of oral nutritional supplements available, their properties and indications for use

Type	Properties	Examples*	Uses/comments
1 kcal/ml milk type sip feed	*Nutritionally complete* 1 kcal/ml Approximate composition per 100 kcal: 4 g protein 3 mmol Na 3 mmol K Ready to drink tetra pack, cup or can presentation Sweet and savoury flavours available ACBS prescribable	Fresubin® Original Drink (Fresenius Kabi) Ensure™ (Abbott) Clinutren Iso® (Nestlé)	Can be used as a supplement or a sole source of nutrition May be preferred by those who find higher energy supplements too rich
High energy 'milk type' sip feed	*Nutritionally complete* 1.5–1.7 kcal/ml Similar composition per 100 kcal as 1 kcal sip feeds (*see above*) Ready to drink usually tetra pack or cup presentation Variety of sweet and savoury flavours ACBS prescribable	Ensure Plus™ (Abbott) Fortisip™ (Nutricia) Fresubin® Energy Drink (Fresenius Kabi) Clinutren® 1.5 (Nestlé) Resource® Shake (Novartis)	Can be used as a supplement or a sole source of nutrition

Type	Composition	Products	Comments
'Juice type' sip feed	*Not nutritionally complete* (no fat and lower levels of several electrolytes) 1.25–1.5 kcal/ml Approximate nutritional composition per 100 kcal: 3 g protein <1 mmol Na <1 mmol K Ready to drink cup or tetra pack presentation ACBS prescribable	Enlive™ (Abbott) Fortijuice™ (Nutricia) Clinutren® Fruit (Nestlé) Providextra® (Fresenius Kabi)	To be used as a supplement *not* as a sole source of nutrition Useful for those who dislike milk type supplements. Can be used as clear fluid Higher carbohydrate content therefore use with caution in those with uncontrolled diabetes
Fibre enriched	*Nutritionally complete* High energy 'milk type' sip feed enriched with fibre. (*See* properties of high energy 'milk type' sip feed) ACBS prescribable	Enrich Plus™ (Abbott) Fortisip Multi Fibre™ (Nutricia) Fresubin® Energy Fibre (Fresenius Kabi) Resource® Fibre (Novartis)	May help improve bowel function, whether diarrhoea or constipation Useful for those requiring a high fibre diet
'Yoghurt style' sip feed	*Nutritionally complete* Properties the same as high energy milk type sip feed Sweet flavours only ACBS prescribable	Ensure Plus Yoghurt Style™ (Abbott) Fortifresh™ (Nutricia)	Can be used as an alternative for those who dislike or have tired of 'milk type' supplements
High protein low electrolyte 'milk type' sip feed	*Nutritionally complete* 1 kcal/ml Approximate composition per 100 kcal: 10 g protein 2.2 mmol Na 1–5.1 mmol K	Fortimel™ (Nutricia) Resource® Protein Extra (Novartis)	Where a higher protein intake is required, e.g. renal patients receiving renal replacement therapy

Table 5.1 (continued)

Type	Properties	Examples*	Uses/comments
High protein milk shake supplement	*Not nutritionally balanced* Constitute powder with milk When made up with full fat milk 1 kcal/ml per 100 kcal provides approximately: 5.5 g protein 0.5 mmol Na 0.5–6.3 mmol K Not prescribable	Build up (Nestlé) Complan (Heinz)	Useful for those who dislike standard milk style supplements. Made with fresh milk therefore some people may find it more palatable
High energy milk shake supplement	*Not nutritionally balanced* Constitute powder with milk When made up with full fat milk 2 kcal/ml per 100 kcal provides approximately: 2 g protein <1 mmol Na 1.8–4.3 mmol K ACBS prescribable	Scandishake (SHS) Calshake™ (Fresenius Kabi)	Useful for those who dislike standard milk style supplements Made with fresh milk therefore some people find it more palatable Useful for those who need high energy
'Pudding type' supplement	*Not nutritionally balanced* Semi-solid supplement 1.25–1.5 kcal/g Nutritional composition per 100 kcal: 2–7 g protein 2.5–5 mmol Na 2.5–5 mmol K ACBS prescribable	Forticrem™ (Nutricia) Formance™ (Abbott) Clinutren® Dessert (Nestlé)	Useful for those on a fluid restricted or altered textured diet and for those who dislike other liquid supplements

Supplement	Description	Examples	Uses
Carbohydrate supplement	*Not nutritionally balanced* Can be liquid or powder – usually maltodextrins or glucose Does not contain protein, fat, vitamins or minerals ACBS prescribable	Maxijul (SHS) Polycal (Nutricia) Polycose (Abbott) Caloreen (Nestlé) Vitajoule (Vitaflo)	Add into drinks or food or the liquid version can be taken on its own Useful for those who need increased energy but are managing adequate vitamins, minerals and protein
Lipid supplement	*Not nutritionally balanced* Lipid emulsions either rich in MCTs or LCTs Do not contain protein or vitamins or minerals	Calogen (LCT) (SHS) Liquigen (MCT) (SHS)	Can be added to food or cooking or taken alone Useful for those who need increased energy but are managing adequate vitamins, minerals and protein MCT supplements can be used to replace ordinary fat in the diet for those who do not tolerate LCT, e.g. severe fat malabsorption, inborn errors of lipid metabolism
Protein supplement	*Not nutritionally balanced* Protein powders. Some also contain carbohydrate	Procal™ (Vitaflo) Maxipro (SHS) Protifar (Nutricia) Promod (Abbott)	Can be added to food and cooking Useful for those who require increased protein but are managing adequate energy, vitamins and minerals

*Examples have been given of some of the common supplements at time of going to print. Check *BNF*, *MIMS*, advisor chart or with individual companies for up-to-date products.
LCT = long chain triglyceride. MCT = medium chain triglyceride.

Enteral tube feeding
Choice of enteral tube feed

There is a wide variety of commercially produced enteral tube feeds for adults (*see* Table 5.2). The choice of feed will depend on:

- the route of nutritional support
- the nutritional requirements of the patient
- the nutritional intake of the patient
- the presence of any gastrointestinal impairment
- the patient's clinical condition, e.g. the presence of renal failure, liver failure.

Broad categories of enteral tube feeds

- *Polymeric feeds*: contain whole protein, carbohydrate and fat.
- Polymeric feeds may have fibre added and may be concentrated. They can be used as a sole source of nutrition for those without any special nutrient requirements.
- Polymeric feeds with increased nutrients are new products designed for those on long-term enteral feeding with low energy requirements. They are nutritionally complete at lower energy levels: 1000–1200 kcal.
- *Pre-digested (elemental and semi-elemental) feeds*: for those with malabsorption.
- *Disease-specific feeds*: the nutrient composition is altered to meet the needs of those with diseases requiring special diets, e.g. renal failure.
- *Immune-modulating or enhancing feeds*: these feeds contain extra substrates which may alter the immune and inflammatory responses. The commonly used substrates are: amino acids glutamine and arginine, RNA, ω-3 fatty acids and anti-oxidants. There is evidence gathering for the use of these products in certain surgical, trauma, critically ill and cancer patients. However, they are still very much at an early stage in terms of clarification of indications for use, and there have been concerns about the safety of these products in some patient groups. The decision to use these products should be made on an individual basis. This should be based on the clinical evidence available for the use of each individual product in the same patient group.

Presentation of enteral tube feeds

Wherever possible closed feeding systems should be used where the feed comes in a sterile pre-filled container and the action of attaching the giving set pierces the container. This type of system has been shown to reduce the risk of bacterial contamination. Every effort should be made to avoid using powdered feeds or decanting feeds, as this practice is associated with a higher incidence of bacterial contamination.

Further reading

- Consensus Recommendations From the US Summit on Immune-Enhancing Enteral Therapy (2001) *JPEN*. **25**: S61–3.
- Talpers SS, Romberger DJ, Bunce SB *et al.* (1992) Nutritionally associated increased carbon dioxide production. Excess total calories *vs* high proportion of carbohydrate calories. *Chest*. **102**: 551–5.

Table 5.2 The main types of enteral tube feeds available for use in adults and their indications for use

Feed type	Properties	Indications/comments
Standard feed	1 kcal/ml Approximate nutritional composition per 100 kcal: 4 g protein 3.5 mmol Na 3.5 mmol K	Used for patients without any special nutrient requirements
High energy	1.5–2 kcal/ml Most provide similar, or slightly lower, nutrient composition per 100 kcal as standard feeds	Those requiring a lower volume, e.g.: fluid restriction overnight feeding high energy requirements where the volume of a standard feed may not be tolerated
Fibre feed	Fibre-enriched versions of standard feeds, high energy feeds and one immune enhanced feed are available Usually mixed source of fibre, soluble and insoluble	Sometimes used as the standard feed May normalise bowel function – either diarrhoea or constipation – and is therefore worth trying if bowel function is troublesome, although hard evidence of efficacy is lacking in the literature
Low energy feed (nutritionally complete)	Nutritionally complete in 1000–1200 kcal Some have fibre added 0.8–1.2 kcal/ml Approximate nutritional composition per 100 kcal: 4.5–5 g protein 4.8–6.3 mmol Na 3.8–6 mmol K	For those on long-term enteral feeding who have lower energy requirements

Table 5.2   (continued)

Feed type	Properties	Indications/comments
High energy/high protein	1.2–1.5 kcal/ml Approximately 5 g of protein per 100 kcal Other nutrient composition similar to standard feeds	High energy and protein requirements, e.g. catabolic patients
Soya	Soya protein instead of milk protein Composition same as standard 1 kcal/ml feeds	Those with cow's milk protein allergy. (Alternatively a peptide or elemental feed could be used, especially if it is not known whether soya protein is tolerated)

High energy/low electrolyte	2 kcal/ml
	Approximate nutritional composition per 100 kcal:
	  3–4 g protein
	  1.5 mmol Na and K
	Also lower in other nutrients, e.g. phosphate, fat soluble vitamins
		Where a low volume but standard protein feed is required, e.g. renal patients on haemodialysis or peritoneal dialysis
		May also be used in other conditions requiring low volume, low electrolyte feed, e.g. liver patients with ascites who require a low volume and low sodium intake
		These feeds were developed for renal patients; therefore if used for other patient groups may need to supplement certain nutrients, e.g. liver patients may need extra phosphate (especially if alcoholic)

High energy/low electrolyte/low protein feed	2 kcal/ml Approximate nutritional composition per 100 kcal: 2 g protein <2.3 mmol Na <2 mmol K	Patients requiring protein, fluid and electrolyte restriction, e.g. renal patients not on renal replacement therapy

	Composition	Uses
Low sodium	Composition as for a standard 1 kcal/ml feed but Na 1.1 mmol/100 ml	Severe sodium restriction, e.g. liver patients with ascites, head injured patients with high intracranial pressure who need to be kept dehydrated
High fat/low carbohydrate	1.5 kcal/ml Nutrient composition per 100 kcal similar to standard feed	Can be helpful in patients with CO_2 retention, e.g. ventilated patients or those with chronic respiratory failure. As high carbohydrate diets further increase CO_2 levels, low carbohydrate diets theoretically can help this situation, although evidence in the literature is lacking
Peptide	Protein is as peptides or a combination of peptides and free amino acids, i.e. requiring less enzymatic digestion Low fat and high protein peptide feeds are available Some are rich in MCTs	Pancreatic insufficiency or malabsorption, where digestive enzymes are lacking Those high in MCTs are useful in severe fat malabsorption, e.g. cystic fibrosis
Elemental	Diets made up of the simple nutrient 'building blocks' Protein as free amino acids Carbohydrate is usually as glucose or maltodextrins ('simpler' molecules and easier to digest than more complex carbohydrates) Low in fat – some are rich in MCTs 0.8 kcal/ml Approximate nutritional composition per 100 kcal: 2.5 g protein 3 mmol Na 3 mmol K	Severe malabsorption Can be used as a liquid diet to treat Crohn's disease (*see* p. 106) although whole protein diets have been found to be as effective Those high in MCTs are useful in severe fat malabsorption, e.g. cystic fibrosis

Table 5.2 (*continued*)

Feed type	Properties	Indications/comments
'Immune modulating' feeds	Enriched with arginine, ω-3 fatty acids and in some cases RNA and/or glutamine Higher protein content due to additional amino acids	May reduce infectious complications in patients undergoing GI surgery and trauma patients (US Consensus 2001 – *see* further reading) In order to be beneficial needs to be given early (preferably pre-operatively in elective surgical patients) and in adequate volumes Should be used with caution in septic patients as may increase mortality
Glutamine enriched	Some feeds are enriched with glutamine or glutamine and other immunonutrients, or glutamine can be added separately	Evidence that enteral glutamine may help reduce the incidence of infections in patients undergoing bone marrow transplantation Some evidence that glutamine reduces infectious complications in the critically ill; however, consensus is still to be achieved

Routes for enteral feeding

Nasogastric feeding

Indications

- Short-term nasogastric (NG) feeding for patients with full use of their stomach without complications such as vomiting or aspiration:
  - impaired swallow, e.g. stroke, motor neurone disease, Parkinson's disease, head injury
  - altered level of consciousness making oral feeding impossible
  - ventilated patients with tracheostomy
  - dysphagia without complete oropharyngeal/oesophageal obstruction, i.e. head and neck and oesophageal cancer.
- Supplement inadequate oral intake:
  - cystic fibrosis
  - hypercatabolic states, e.g. burn injury, decompensated liver disease
  - facial injury
  - HIV wasting
  - psychological/psychiatric reasons, e.g. anorexia nervosa.
- Occasionally for long-term feeding where alternative methods are either unsafe or against patient preference.

Contraindications

- Obstructive pathology in oropharynx or oesophagus preventing passage of tube.
- Gastric outflow obstruction:
  - mechanical, e.g. pyloric ulceration/stricture, tumour
  - functional gastroparesis, as seen in critical care setting (*see* p. 92) or diabetes.
- Intestinal obstruction:
  - mechanical, i.e. obstructing small intestinal pathology
  - ileus.
- Intestinal perforation.
- Proximal gastrointestinal tract fistula.
- Facial injury.

Practical considerations

What tube to use

There are two main types of NG feeding tubes: fine bore and wide bore (e.g. Ryles). Wide bore tubes should not be sited specifically for enteral feeding (*see* Table 5.3). They may be used in the short term if there are concerns about poor gastric emptying and increased risk of aspiration. This is relevant mainly for critically ill patients and should be discussed with the dietitian and medical team.

  NB: *Nasal feeding tubes should never be passed on patients with basal skull fractures as the tube may be malpositioned and enter the brain. In these cases tubes may be passed orogastrically, i.e.* via *the mouth to the stomach under the advice of the medical team.*

Care of an NG tube

(i) How to pass an NG tube. (*See* Table 5.4.) Local policy/protocols, where they exist, should be referred to. Placing an NG tube can be a distressing procedure. Careful patient preparation is vital to provide reassurance and to increase compliance. If there is difficulty in placing the tube do *not* allow the patient to become distressed by repeated attempts. The urgency for placing the tube should

Table 5.3   Comparison of fine bore and wide bore NG tubes

	Fine bore	*Wide bore*
Size	6–9 FG (French Gauge)	9–22 FG
Material	Polyurethane	Polyvinyl chloride
Use	Enteral feeding	Stomach aspiration and drainage
Advantages	Soft material, patient usually becomes unaware of tube within a few hours of insertion Patient can eat and drink normally (if appropriate)	Easy to aspirate stomach contents
Disadvantages	May not be able to aspirate large amounts from stomach – *see* section below, on aspirating from fine bore tubes	May cause ulceration of oesophageal and nasal tissue, is hard and uncomfortable, may limit patient's solid food intake
Ideal time *in situ*	7 days–6 months	3–5 days
Cost (approx)	£6.00	£0.26

be reviewed and, if required, a further attempt to insert the tube should occur once the patient has recovered, and given consent to continue. Only verbal consent is required for this procedure.

(ii) Verification of correct tube position. (*See* Table 5.5.) Ward-based staff are responsible for confirming that NG tubes are correctly positioned, both on insertion and during subsequent use. It is crucial to differentiate between gastric and respiratory placement to prevent pulmonary complications.

There are many methods to test tube position, few of which are evidence based. Although radiological confirmation is the 'gold standard' it is expensive, disruptive and frequently leads to delays in starting feeding regimens. Auscultation (putting air down the tube) is not a reliable method of predicting tube placement, as differentiation between stomach, oesophagus or respiratory tract cannot be made accurately. This is no longer considered to be acceptable practice.

The method of choice for verifying correct tube placement is pH testing of tube aspirate. This is safe, accurate and cost-effective. Litmus paper is not sufficiently sensitive to distinguish between degrees of acidity, e.g. gastric aspirate has a pH < 4 and bronchial secretions a pH > 6. A more sensitive pH indicator strip should be used.

(iii) When should tube position be checked? It is quite common for fine bore feeding tubes to become dislodged without the staff being aware, e.g. the tube tip can spontaneously migrate into the oesophagus, leaving the patient at risk of regurgitation and aspiration.

Table 5.4 Insertion of an NG tube. (Refer to local policy/protocols if available)

Equipment required

Appropriate sized fine bore tube	pH indicator paper
Glass of water and straw (if able to swallow)	Receiver
Sterile water or sodium chloride 0.9%	Tissues
5 ml syringe for fine bore, or bladder-tipped syringe for wide bore tube	Stethoscope
	Lubricating jelly
Non-sterile latex gloves and disposable plastic apron	Hypoallergenic tape and scissors

Intervention	Rationale
Ideally this procedure should take place during the daytime	To prevent distressing the patient at nighttime and to ensure support is easily available
Explain procedure and rationale of NG feeding tube to the patient	To gain informed consent and co-operation from the patient. Document this
If possible assist the patient into an upright position using pillows if needed or on their side if they are unable to be upright	To ease the insertion of the NG tube and to reduce the risk of gastric aspiration if reflux occurs
Ask the patient about nasal blockages, breaks, fractures, polyps or previous surgery to the nose. Also ask if patient has preference and ask the patient which nostril to use – consider which side they sleep on, e.g. which side has been affected by their stroke	To ensure patient involvement and choice and to optimise comfort and compliance once tube has been placed
Ask the patient to blow their nose	Clear the nasal passages
Measure the length from the patient's ear lobe to the bridge of the nose, plus the distance from the bridge of the nose to the xiphisternum (approx 50–65 cm)	To provide estimate of length to which tube should be inserted

Table 5.4 (continued)

Intervention	Rationale
Arrange with the patient a signal by which he/she can stop the proceedings if so desired	To gain patient's confidence and enable the patient to take control if procedure becomes distressing
Wash hands and put on non-sterile latex gloves and disposable plastic apron	Universal precautions
If fine bore tube: ensure guide wire is firmly anchored in tube and flush with 10 ml water or sodium chloride. Dip end of tube in water. Extra lubricating jelly can be used if necessary	To activate hydromer coating and provide lubrication
If the patient is able to swallow safely give him/her the glass of water ± straw to make sipping easier	Check/assess the ability to swallow prior to beginning the procedure
Introduce the tube into the chosen nostril and gently slide it backwards approx 15 cm	To introduce the tube as far as the pharynx
Ask the patient to put his/her chin on his/her chest, take a sip of water, and hold the water in his/her mouth. Ask the patient to swallow. As he/she swallows advance the tube 10–15 cm and stop	To assist the tube entering the oesophagus and not the trachea
If the patient shows signs of distress, e.g. coughing, gasping or breathlessness, remove the tube immediately	Suggests the tube has entered the trachea
If the patient is calm with no signs of distress continue to advance the tube whilst the patient sips and swallows water, until the required length has been passed	Safe to continue
If the tube proves difficult to pass despite repeated attempts, stop and allow the patient at least an hour to recover. Review need for alternative hydration with medical team	Prevent distressing patient but ensure adequate fluid intake is maintained

Action	Rationale
If successful placement, temporarily secure the tube to cheek or nose with hypoallergenic tape, ensuring it is comfortable	The position of the NG tube needs to be confirmed prior to securing it firmly
Confirm correct position of tube – *see* (ii) below and Table 5.5	
Following confirmation of correct placement of the tube, mark the tube where it leaves the patient's nose using a permanent pen unless the tube has markings making this unnecessary	To provide guide if the tube moves
If fine bore tube: remove the guide wire using gentle traction *NB: Once guide wire has been removed this must not be replaced whilst the tube is still in the patient*	Feeding cannot commence with wire *in situ*
Firmly secure the tube on the nose or cheek using hypoallergenic tape	To avoid discomfort and pressure sores ensure that the tube is not resting against the edge of the nostril. Confirm comfortable position with patient
Discuss the risks of accidentally removing the NG tube with the patient and methods of avoiding this	To increase patient understanding and co-operation
Document procedure, actions and findings in patient's record	Provide ongoing evaluation and in accordance with requirements for record keeping and documentation

Table 5.5 Method for verifying correct tube placement. (Refer to local policy/ protocols if available)

Action	Rationale
If the patient is allowed to swallow to assist insertion, give only water	Other fluids, particularly fruit juices, will alter pH
Insert 10 ml of air into the tube using a 20 ml syringe	To clear the tube of any debris and to move the tip of the tube away from the gastric mucosa
Withdraw aspirate using a > 20 ml syringe. Less than 1 ml of aspirate is sufficient	To obtain aspirate for testing
Apply aspirate to pH strip and compare colour bars to those on the pH scale	A reading of $pH < 4$ indicates gastric placement
Flush tube with ∼30 ml water	To clear tube of aspirated fluid
If unable to achieve aspirate arrange X-ray	

Therefore tube position should be checked at the following times.

- On initial placement.
- Before each bolus feed or when starting up a feed.
- Before giving medication only if tube not currently used.
- Following vomiting or violent coughing.
- If the tube is accidentally dislodged.
- If the patient complains of discomfort.

The presence of enteral feed in the stomach will affect the gastric pH. If you need to check the pH whilst the feed is running you will need to stop the feed for at least 30 minutes.

NB. pH testing will only help assess the position of the tip of the tube at the time it is tested. Nursing staff should continue to monitor the patient for clinical signs of tube malposition, such as coughing, retching, vomiting and increasing respiratory distress not explained by any other cause.

Feed administration
(i) Patient positioning for feeding. Patients should be fed at a 30–45° upright angle unless medically contraindicated, e.g. spinal injury. They should not be fed lying flat nor do they need to be fed while sitting bolt upright at 90°. It is advisable not to lie flat until an hour after the feed otherwise reflux or regurgitation may occur.

(ii) Method of feeding. *Pump feeding.* This is a continuous infusion, usually at a rate between 80–100 ml/hr depending on the patient requirements.
Gravity feeding. This is where a large (50–60 ml) syringe is filled and attached to a giving set and then held higher than the patient. The contents of the syringe

then flow into the patient over 10–20 minutes. This method of 'bolus' feeding avoids long periods of time 'attached' to a pump, and is popular with some. There has been concern that it is associated with a higher risk of complication, such as aspiration, abdominal bloating and discomfort, although this has not been adequately tested in clinical trials.

At present, the choice between pump feeding or gravity feeding will depend on local practice and resources.

(iii) Feeding duration. When pump feeding, it is usually not necessary to feed for the full 24 hour duration; 16–18 hours a day is usually sufficient to give the required amount of feed. This gives the patient 6–8 hours free of feeding, which can either be in the daytime or at night, depending on what arrangements suit the patient and carers/nursing staff best.

Complications
- Removal by patient.
    - Purposeful: consider patient withdrawal of consent.
    - Confused: may need re-siting or, if repeated removal, consider either means of restraint (*see* Chapter 12) or alternative means of nutritional support, e.g. percutaneous endoscopic gastrostomy (PEG), *see* below.
- Oesophageal ulceration/strictures: now uncommon if fine bore tubes are used for the short term.

Table 5.6 Management of a blocked tube. (Refer to local policy/protocols if available)

Intervention	Rationale
Tubes should be flushed with at least 50 ml cooled boiled or sterile water pre- and post-feeds and medication. It is particularly important to flush the tube before a rest period	To prevent blockage
If the tube is not being used it should be flushed daily with at least 50 ml of water	To ensure the tube remains patent
If the tube blocks using a 30/50 ml syringe, flush with 20–50 ml warm water If available fizzy drink, such as mineral water, can be used Pancreatic enzymes, e.g. Pancrex V or creon, can be prescribed and put down the tube. After 60 minutes patency can be assessed	To unblock the tube and so prevent unnecessary tube replacement
Document all actions and findings in patient's record	To provide ongoing communication and in accordance with standards for record keeping and documentation

- Malposition into the lungs can lead to infection, effusion and empyema. Occasionally the tube can be malpositioned intracranially. With appropriate means of verification (*see* above) this should not happen.
- Blockage (*see* Table 5.6): all types of enteral feeding tubes may become blocked and the fine bore tubes are particularly at risk from this. This problem is avoidable if the tube is flushed with water before starting and after completion of a feed, 4–6 hourly throughout feeding and before and after medication, as residue can quickly build up. All types of tube can be unblocked using the methods described; soda water may unblock tubes and certain enzymes in pineapple juice break down the solidified feed. Acidic fizzy drinks, such as cola, can coagulate protein in the tube and exacerbate the problem – these should therefore not be used.

Nasojejunal feeding
Indications
- Nasojejunal (NJ) feeding is used for short-term access for patients with a functioning gastrointestinal tract but in whom the stomach needs to be bypassed, i.e. where there is a gastric outflow obstruction (*see* under NG tube contraindications).
- Pancreatitis (*see* p. 91).
- Risk of aspiration with intragastric feeding.

There are two types of NJ tube.

1 Single lumen. This can be placed with or without an endoscope.
2 Double lumen. This has an additional gastric aspiration port, which needs to be placed endoscopically, radiologically or during surgery.

Contraindications
As per NG feeding contraindications (*see* above).

Practical considerations
- *See* Table 5.7.
- Some tubes are designed to pass spontaneously into the duodenum, such as the Bengmark tube (Nutricia, UK). Where gastric motility is normal, trans-pyloric passage should be achievable in 70–80%, especially if a bolus of a pro-motility agent such as metoclopramide is given concurrently. In the atonic stomach trans-pyloric passage cannot be relied upon and alternative means of securing post-pyloric feeding should be sought.
- Weighted tubes have no advantage over unweighted tubes, and they probably have a higher incidence of retrograde passage back into the stomach. There is therefore no indication for their use.
- Most NJ tubes require endoscopic placement, which can be technically demanding. If the distal end of the tube is not placed beyond the duodeno–jejunal flexure or Ligament of Treitz (*see* Figure 5.2) there will invariably be retrograde passage of the tube back into the stomach.
- Plain abdominal X-ray is required to verify placement, unless placed under screening.

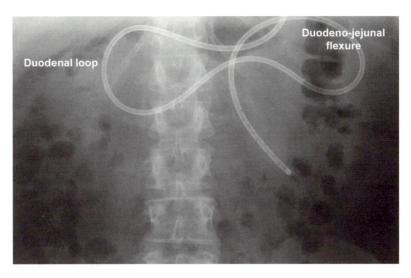

Figure 5.2 Nasojejunal tube *in situ*.

Complications
As per NG tube complications.

Percutaneous endoscopically-placed gastrostomy tube
There are a number of different types of PEG tube in terms of size (9–24 FG), internal fixator (flange, balloon) and material (*see* Figure 5.3a). In addition there are 'button' gastrostomies (*see* Figure 5.3b) that are more cosmetically acceptable, especially for the younger patient. They all work on the same principle but nevertheless familiarisation with the specific type that is stocked in a particular hospital will be useful.

Indications
PEG is a longer-term route of feeding for those with a functioning gastrointestinal tract who are either unable to eat/swallow or whose oral intake is inadequate (*see* NG indications, above).

Contraindications
• Absolute.
  – Inability to pass endoscope due to obstructing pathology in oropharynx or oesophagus.*
  – Obstructing gastric outflow pathology.
• Relative.
  – Severe obesity (due to technical difficulties accessing the stomach).*
  – Uncorrected coagulopathy.
  – Portal hypertension.
  – Active gastric ulceration/malignancy.
  – Gastroparesis.
  – Gastrectomy (total or partial).*

Table 5.7   Care of the patient receiving NJ or jejunostomy feeding. (Refer to local policy/protocols if available)

Feeding	
Action	Rationale
Feeding can be started in the early post-operative period at the discretion and instruction of the nutrition team, surgical or medical team managing the patient	The site of upper GI surgery is bypassed as is any delayed gastric emptying
Only use the regimen prescribed by the dietitian	Specialised feeds may be required if there are digestion/absorption problems
Start the feed at a slow rate and increase cautiously as stated on the dietetic regimen	The jejunum is a smaller reservoir than the stomach therefore the feed rate must be increased slowly
Feeding can be over 24 hours	The jejunum is not an acid environment therefore there is no need for a gap in feeding to allow acidity to return, as is the normal practice with gastric feeding
Always wash hands, wear non-sterile gloves and an apron when setting up the feed or manipulating the tube	Clean procedure must always be used as the defence mechanism of the acidic stomach is bypassed and there is a greater risk of infection

Tube care	
Action	Rationale
Ensure that NJ tube is fixed securely to the nose and/or cheek so as not to interfere with the field of vision	To avoid displacement as NJ tubes need to be replaced endoscopically. Taped by the side of the face will not be uncomfortable for the patient
Make an indelible mark on the tube at the point where it exits the nose. If the tube moves do not feed; contact the doctor or appropriate nurse, e.g. nutrition nurse, to review	In order to detect if tube has moved. If the tube has moved its position may need to be checked with X-ray
Ensure that the jejunostomy is secured in place with sutures for the first 7 days and steristrips thereafter	Jejenostomy tubes often do not have a retention device and need to be secured
Flush the tube every 6 hours with 30 ml of sterile water using a 50 ml syringe	To prevent blockage. Jejunal tubes are narrower and/or longer, therefore are at more risk of blocking. Do not use a syringe smaller than 50 ml as the pressure will be too great and the tube may split

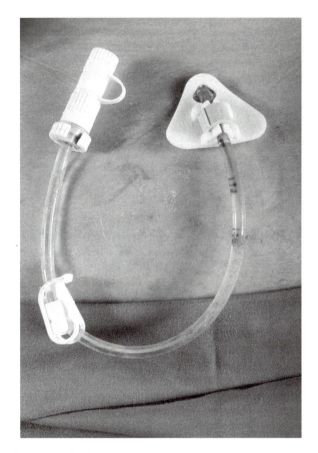

Figure 5.3a   Percutaneous gastrostomy.

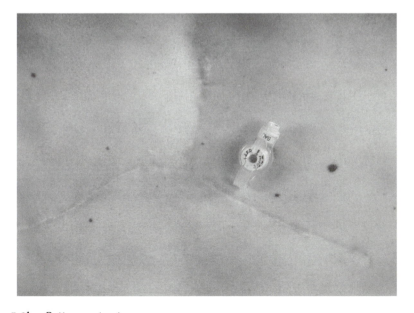

Figure 5.3b   Button gastrostomy.

– Severe kyphoscoliosis (may be difficult to access stomach).*
– Current peritoneal dialysis.

*May be achievable if done under radiological guidance to locate stomach (radiologically-inserted gastrostomy or RIG).

Practical considerations
- Insertion of a PEG is not without morbidity and mortality, especially in elderly, frail patients with significant co-morbidity.
- Patient selection is very important (*see* ethics, Chapter 12).
- There are button gastrostomies that are cosmetically more acceptable, especially for the younger patient (*see* Figure 5.3b).

PEG insertion
- Technique for insertion is discussed elsewhere (*see* further reading list).
- Insertion is not a sterile procedure, but current UK guidelines recommend it is done with antibiotic prophylaxis, such as cefotaxime 2 g or co-amoxyclav 2.2 g given 30 minutes prior to the procedure (British Society of Gastroenterology, 2001 – *see* further reading list).
- Feeding can be commenced 6 hours after the procedure as per the feeding regimen drawn up by a dietitian.

PEG care
See Tables 5.8 and 5.9 for details of immediate care following PEG tube insertion and ongoing care for tubes.

PEG removal
- If the PEG is removed within 2–3 weeks of insertion a formal tract will not have formed, with consequent risk of spillage of gastric contents into the peritoneal cavity leading to peritonitis. This also means that it will not be possible to re-insert a feeding tube down the same tract as it will not find its way into the gastric lumen. Therefore if the PEG does come out in the first few weeks of insertion, whether at the hand of the patient or through some other mishap, the stoma site should be covered, antibiotic cover instituted and, if nutritional support is still required, an alternative access, e.g. NG tube, used until the wound has healed.
- After 2–3 weeks a formal fistulous tract will have formed and if the tube is then removed there will be no risk of peritonitis/sepsis. However, this tract will close over within 4–6 hours. Therefore, if it comes out accidentally a replacement will need re-insertion immediately. Ideally this should be a fresh PEG or button, but could be a balloon gastrostomy, a Foley catheter, or equivalent, that can be a temporary replacement for up to several days until a PEG can be formally replaced.
- Elective removal is usually done endoscopically. An alternative, which avoids endoscopy, is cutting the tube close to the skin and allowing the internal fixator to pass spontaneously through the gastrointestinal tract. There are no reported incidents of obstruction, e.g. at the ileocaecal junction, and this method is probably safe.

Complications
The following are complications which may arise (common complications are in italics).

- Early.
  - *Pain*:
    - (i)   usually within first 24 hours
    - (ii)   treat with simple analgesia
    - (iii) if severe exclude peritonitis/tube displacement into anterior abdominal wall.

Table 5.8   Immediate care following PEG tube insertion. (Refer to local policy/ protocols if available)

Action	Rationale
The patient should remain nil by tube for 6 hours after insertion Patients who are allowed to take oral intake also need to remain nil by mouth for 6 hours	Endoscopic procedures can cause gastroparesis and therefore delay gastric emptying Swallow may be affected while sedation is wearing off
Temperature, pulse, respiratory rate and blood pressure must be monitored post procedure: half-hourly for 4 hours hourly for 2 hours qds thereafter or as appropriate for the underlying clinical condition	Post procedure observations must be conducted as the patient has undergone an invasive procedure under sedation Potential complications such as bleeding, hypotension and respiratory depression can be detected early, monitored, recorded and acted upon
The site under the gastrostomy fixation device should be inspected for any blood or serous fluid leakage. If leakage present, a further key-hole dressing should be applied using an aseptic technique. If bleeding does not stop or becomes worse then a member of the medical staff must be informed	The gastrostomy site must be monitored post procedure as there is a risk of bleeding post procedure Further dressings/assessment/suturing may be required
After 6 hours the PEG tube can be flushed with water Liaise with the dietitian about the feeding regimen	The gastrostomy tube requires regular flushing to keep it patent The dietitian will decide an appropriate feeding regimen for the patient and when this should commence
Patient position (unless contraindicated) must be at 30–45° when water/ feeding starts	This will prevent reflux of feed which can lead to aspiration/inhalation
Maintain accurate observation and fluid balance chart	To assess post procedure condition and to monitor fluid balance when feed has commenced

- Haemorrhage: unusual if clotting screen within normal limits. As malnutrition can lead to vitamin K deficiency, the prothrombin time/INR should always be checked prior to procedure.
- Peritonitis.
- Pneumoperitoneum: it should be noted that there will always be some free after PEG insertion.
- Gastrocolic fistula: due to interposition of colon between anterior abdominal wall and stomach.
- Late.
  - *Stoma infection*:
    (i)   attention to proper stoma care (*see* above and/or local policy)
    (ii) take swabs from stoma
    (iii) course of appropriate antibiotics, e.g. flucloxacillin, erythromycin
    (iv) not necessary to remove PEG or stop feeding unless severe ulceration or wound breakdown.
  - *Tube blockage*:
    (i) always flush with water before and after each feed/medication (*see* above)
    (ii) if blocked use sodium bicarbonate solution or diluted pancreatic enzyme.
  - *Aspiration*: can be minimised by feeding for no more than 20 hours per day at an elevation of at least 30°.
  - Buried bumper: internal fixator migrates into gastric/anterior abdominal wall leading to tube blockage. This usually requires surgery to remove.
  - Tumour tract seeding: a few case reports of PEGs inserted into patients with oropharyngeal or oesophageal tumours developing neoplastic seeding in stoma tracts. Where the PEG is inserted as part of palliative care, this is unlikely to be of relevance in the patient's life-time.
  - Overgranulation:
    (i) can occur at stoma site and bleed/become painful
    (ii) steroid cream or silver nitrate can usually deal with it.

Percutaneous endoscopically-placed jejunostomy tube
Indications
Indications for percutaneous endoscopically-placed jejunostomy (PEJ) tube are as per NJ indications (*see* above), but where longer-term access is required.

Contraindications
As for PEG contraindications (*see* above).

Practical considerations
- Insertion technique similar to that of a PEG, except that a direct puncture into the small intestine is required. It can be difficult to achieve adequate trans-illumination or indentation on finger pressure to the external abdominal wall. A few endoscopists are ardent protagonists of this technique, but most will not undertake this procedure preferring a surgically-placed jejunostomy or jejunal extension to PEG (*see* below).
- Care of tubes and management of feeding regimens as per NJ (*see* above).

Complications
As per PEG complications (*see* above).

Table 5.9   Ongoing care for PEG tubes. (Refer to local policy/protocols if available)

Intervention	Rationale
Offer support and guidance	To ensure patient understanding
Offer 4 hourly mouth care to patients who are unable to attend to this independently or who are nil by mouth	To provide comfort and minimise the risk of Candida or other mouth infections
Position the patient (unless contraindicated) at a minimum of 30° when feeding starts	This will prevent reflux of feed which can lead to pulmonary aspiration
Flush gastrostomy tube with 30–50 ml sterile water before and after each feed	To prevent the tube from becoming blocked. (Check patient is not on a fluid restriction)
Give the feed according to dietetic advice/ prescription	The type of feed and the amount to be infused are specific to the patient
Stop the feed at least 30 minutes before chest physiotherapy	Minimises the risk of reflux of feed which can lead to pulmonary aspiration
Maintain an accurate fluid balance chart	To assess fluid balance and ensure the prescribed volume of feed is being delivered
Check the blood sugar at the outset, and do a daily urinalysis	Enteral feeds contain glucose and therefore blood sugar can be raised when feeds are first started
Ensure weight is checked on a regular basis	Assessment of fluid balance and nutrition
If the patient has an impaired swallow, or develops one, ensure that a referral is made to the speech and language therapist	To reassess the swallow and ability to manage oral foods and fluids
The gastrostomy site should remain dressed for 7–10 days and then can be left exposed if healed	To allow the wound to heal and prevent cross-infection from other sources
Do not use Opsite or bulky dressings to external disc/flange. Position flange slightly away from wound site	Bulky dressings may cause excess pressure and risk a pressure ulcer under the flange
Rotate tube 360° daily	To prevent blanching
For balloon gastrostomies (in addition to the above): every week, check the balloon is inflated with the amount of water as stated on the inflation port. Refill as required	To ensure the tube is firmly held in place
The external flange should be close to the skin so that the gastrostomy tube cannot move in or out during the first month. However, it should not be so tight that it causes discomfort or pressure necrosis. After a month the tension can be relaxed	The tension ensures that the stomach wall is pulled right up to the anterior abdominal wall and prevents intraperitoneal leakage until healing has taken place
Check the site daily for redness, inflammation or discharge. If a discharge is present, obtain a swab for microbiology, clean the site with sterile saline and apply a dry dressing	To detect, prevent and treat skin irritation or site infection

Jejunal extension to PEG

Jejunal extensions to PEG (PEGJ) are commercially available 'extensions' that attach to the PEG and, under endoscopic control, are passed into the duodenum, ideally beyond the duodeno–jejunal flexure.

Indications

As per NJ indications (*see* above), but where longer-term access is required.

Contraindications

As for PEG contraindications (*see* above).

Practical considerations

- PEGJ are fiddly to insert and the attachments at the PEG can be confusing, especially to uninitiated ward staff.
- Long-term success, in terms of maintaining position in the small intestine, is debatable and there is probably no advantage of these over a surgically-placed jejunostomy except in a patient who is too unfit to have a general anaesthetic.
- Care of tubes and management of feeding regimens as per NJ (*see* above).

Complications

- As per PEG complications (*see* above).
- Tube displacement back into stomach requiring re-siting.

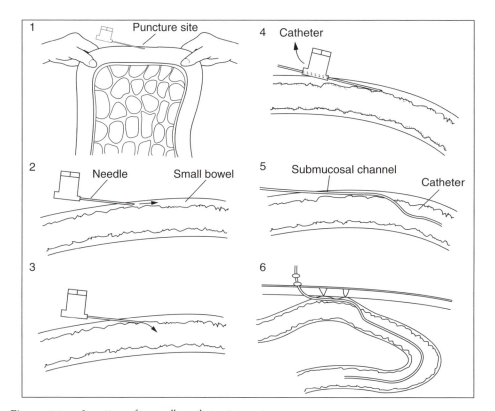

Figure 5.4a Insertion of a needle catheter jejunostomy.

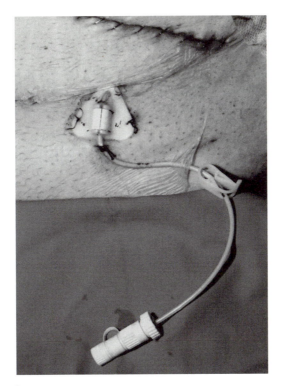

Figure 5.4b Surgical jejunostomy.

Surgically-placed jejunostomy
See Figures 5.4a and 5.4b.

Indications
- As per NJ indications (*see* above), but where longer-term access is required.
- Peri-operative placement to aid post-operative feeding (*see* peri-operative nutrition, Chapter 6).

Contraindications
- Absolute.
  - Jejunal disease, e.g. Crohn's disease or radiation enteritis at the insertion site.
  - Obstructing distal pathology.
- Relative.
  - Ascites.
  - Portal hypertension.
  - Peritoneal dialysis.

Practical considerations
- The best tubes appear to be commercially available needle jejunostomies. They allow for sub-serosal tunnelling and may reduce the risk of leakage. Their disadvantage is perhaps that they tend to be fine bore and as such may block with greater frequency if poorly managed.
- Use of other tubes such as Foley catheter is not ideal, as these are prone to leakage and do not connect easily with enteral feeding equipment.
- Purse string sutures and serosal tunnelling can be used to minimise leakage.

- Care should be taken to approximate and secure the peritoneal and bowel entry sites with serosal and peritoneal stitches. This may again prevent leakage and potential tube kinking and blockage.
- Care of tubes and management of feeding regimens as per NJ (*see* above).

Complications
- Early.
  - *Pain.*
    (i)   Usually not separable from pain of the definitive procedure.
    (ii) Treat with appropriate analgesia.
    (iii) Care should be taken to exclude other post-operative problems.
  - *Haemorrhage.* Rarely the site of post-operative haemorrhage, both intraperitoneal and intraluminal.
  - *Peritonitis.* Leakage around site of luminal contents or feed may lead to peritonitis.
- Late.
  - *Entry site infection.* As for PEG (*see* above).
  - *Tube blockage.* As for PEG (*see* above).

Further reading

- American Society for Gastrointestinal Endoscopy (1998) Role of PEG/PEJ in enteral feeding. *Gastrointest Endosc.* **48**: 699–701.
- British Society of Gastroenterology (2001) *Guidelines in Gastroenterology: antibiotic prophylaxis in gastrointestinal endoscopy.* BSG, London.
- Burnham SP (2000) A guide to naso-gastric tube insertion. *Nursing Times.* **96**(8): 6–7.
- Campos AC and Marchesini JB (1999) Recent advances in the placement of tubes for enteral nutrition. *Curr Opin Clin Nutr Metab Care.* **2**: 265–9.
- DiSario J, Baskin W, Brown R *et al.* (2002) Endoscopic approaches to enteral nutritional support. *Gastrointest Endosc.* **55**: 901–8.
- Dormann AJ and Huchzermeyer H (2002) Endoscopic techniques for enteral nutrition: standards and innovations. *Dig Dis.* **20**: 145–53.
- Fan AC, Baron TH, Rumalla A *et al.* (2002) Comparison of direct percutaneous endoscopic jejunostomy and PEG with jejunal extension. *Gastrointest Endosc.* **56**: 890–4.
- Gopalan S and Khanna S (2003) Enteral nutrition delivery technique. *Curr Opin Clin Nutr Metab Care.* **6**: 313–17.
- Kirby DF, Delegge MH and Fleming CR (1995) American Gastroenterological Association technical review on tube feeding for enteral nutrition. *Gastroenterology.* **108**: 1282–301.
- Metheny N, Wehrle M, Wiersema L *et al.* (1998) Testing feeding tube placement. Auscultation *versus* pH method. *Am J Nurs.* **98**: 37–43.
- Payne KM, King TM and Eisenach JB (1991) The technique of percutaneous endoscopic gastrostomy. A safe and cost-effective alternative to operative gastrostomy. *J Crit Illn.* **6**: 611–19.
- Pearce CB and Duncan HD (2002) Enteral feeding. Nasogastric, nasojejunal, percutaneous endoscopic gastrostomy, or jejunostomy: its indications and limitations. *Postgrad Med J.* **78**: 198–204.

- Safadi B, Marks J and Ponsky J (1998) Percutaneous endoscopic gastrostomy: an update. *Endoscopy.* **30**: 781–9.
- Schurink CA, Tuynman H, Scholten P *et al.* (2001) Percutaneous endoscopic gastrostomy: complications and suggestions to avoid them. *Eur J Gastroenterol Hepatol.* **13**: 819–23.
- Sharma V and Howden C (2000) Meta-analysis of randomized, controlled trials of antibiotic prophylaxis before percutaneous endoscopic gastrostomy. *Am J Gastroenterol.* **95**: 3133–6.
- Shike M and Latkany L (1998) Direct percutaneous endoscopic jejunostomy. *Gastrointest Endosc Clin N Am.* **8**: 569–80.

Drug administration *via* an enteral feeding tube

- Drug administration *via* an enteral feeding tube is an unlicensed use (*see* Figure 5.5) of a licensed medicine.
- Prescribers, pharmacists and nurses must be aware that they are professionally accountable for any adverse effects resulting from the use of this route of administration.
- Consideration should be given to administration of the drug *via* an alternative, licensed route, e.g. rectal, parenteral.
- It is important to consider factors associated with the tube itself, the drug and the method of administration.

Enteral feeding tube considerations
- Tube size and especially tube bore.
- Placement site in the gastrointestinal tract.

Drug therapy considerations
- Pharmacists must be consulted when drugs are to be administered *via* an enteral feeding tube. A full medication review must be undertaken to optimise drug therapy regimen.
- Drugs must not be added to enteral feeds.
- Site of drug absorption, which is a particular problem with jejunal feeding.
- Also consider drug osmolalities – avoid hyperosmolar loads directly into jejunum.
- Drugs/feed interactions may occur (*see* drug–nutrient interactions, p. 81).
- Simplified dosage regimen, i.e. once daily if possible.
- Choice of suitable drug form, i.e. liquid, soluble tablet, injection, or therapeutic substitution to alternative drug available in a suitable form.
- Avoid enteric coated, controlled-release and modified-release preparations.
- Sorbitol content of liquid medicines.
- Do not crush cytotoxic drugs, hormones or steroids due to health risks for the handler.

Drug administration considerations
- Minimise exposure to crushed tablets/capsule contents by wearing gloves.
- Check local policy for use of tap or sterile water.
- An oral, enteral or catheter tipped syringe should be used where possible to minimise the risk of administration *via* the wrong route, i.e. IV.

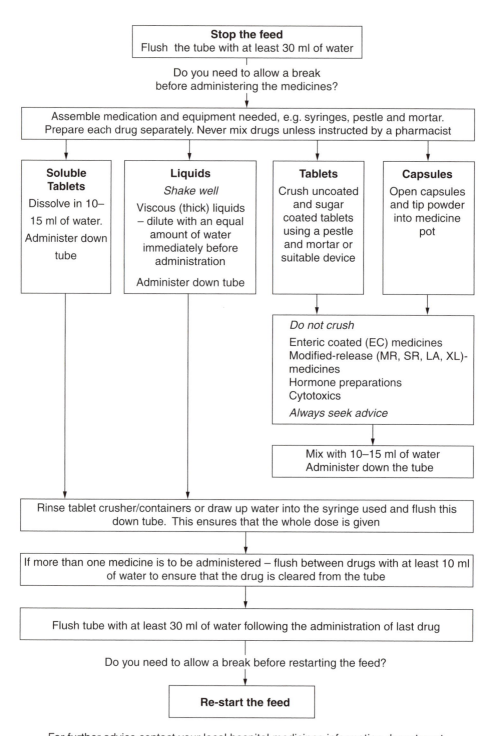

Figure 5.5 Drug administration *via* feeding tubes (refer to local policy/protocols if available).

- A large syringe (50 ml) should be used as a smaller syringe may produce too much pressure and split the tube. Check local policy.
- Some drugs may interact with the feed and need to be administered during a break in the feeding regimen.
- Ensure tube is flushed before and after administration of each drug.
- Tube blockage may occur due to viscosity of liquid preparations; thick liquids may need to be diluted prior to administration. Seek advice.
- Crushed tablets or capsule contents may also cause tube blockage – get advice.
- If tube is blocked, seek specialist advice.
- Use flow chart attached (Figure 5.5).
- If breaks in the feeding regimen are required to administer drugs the dietitian should be consulted to ensure that the quantity of feed delivered is not compromised.

Further reading

- BAPEN working party (2003) *Drug Administration* via *Enteral Feeding Tubes*. BAPEN, Maidenhead.
- Beckwith M, Barton R and Graves C (1997) Guide to drug therapy in patients with enteral feeding tubes: dosage form selection and administration methods. *Hosp Pharmacist*. **32**: 57–64.
- Engle K and Hannawa T (1999) Techniques for administering oral medications to critical care patients receiving continous enteral nutrition. *Am J Health-Syst Pharm*. **56**: 1441–4.
- Thomson F, Naysmith M and Lindsay A (2000) Managing drug therapy in patients receiving enteral and parenteral nutrition. *Hosp Pharmacist*. **7**: 155–64.

Complications of enteral feeding

- On the whole enteral tube feeding is safe.
- Complications relating to enteral feeding itself are:
  - diarrhoea
  - constipation
  - vomiting/aspiration/reflux
  - metabolic complications
  - vitamin/trace element deficiencies.
- Complications related to the tubes and routes of feeding are dealt with in the section, routes for enteral feeding. *See* above.

Diarrhoea
- Common. Affects 10–20% patients on general wards and up to 60% on the intensive care unit.
- Many different definitions in the literature. Pragmatically can be defined as 'loose stools sufficient to inconvenience patient and/or nursing/medical staff'.
- Other disease-related pathology needs to be excluded, e.g. infection, colitis/ enteritis, malabsorption, gut motility disorder.
- Exclude infection, e.g. *Clostridium difficile* – send stool sample.

- Most frequent explanation is medication, e.g. antibiotics, laxatives and drugs formulated with sorbitol, such as aminophylline (sorbitol has a similar effect to lactulose). Where possible these need to be stopped or altered.
- Feeding-related diarrhoea can be associated with:
  - contaminated feeds:
    - (i)   ensure clean technique to set diet up
    - (ii) use sterile 'closed' feeding systems where possible
    - (iii) minimise manipulation of feeding system
    - (iv) keep feed container hanging time to a minimum (no more than 24 hours)
    - (v)   gastric acid will destroy most infused bacteria
    - (vi) acid-suppressing medication may need reviewing in afflicted patients.
  - ↓ albumin:
    - (i) probably leads to gut oedema
    - (ii) the cause of the low albumin, e.g. sepsis, should be addressed.
- Management shown in Figure 5.6.

Constipation
- Usually due to a combination of inadequate fluid, dehydration, poor mobility and drugs (e.g. opiates).
- Ensure no other explanation such as colonic pathology.
- Constipation needs addressing in the usual way with laxatives/suppositories etc.
- Fibre feeds can help and are usually worth trying.

Vomiting/aspiration/reflux
- Both NG and PEG feeding can increase the risk of aspiration. Both can interfere with gastro-oesophageal sphincter function, and wide bore NG tubes do so more than fine bore tubes. The former therefore should be avoided.
- Where possible patients should be fed at 30–45°.
- Try standard anti-emetics and prokinetic agents.
- If bolus feeding, change to continuous pump-assisted feeding.
- If pump feeding, ↓ rate and use high energy, lower volume feeds.
- Where there is a significant problem with functional gastric hold-up, consider post-pyloric feeding (*see* above, routes for enteral feeding).

Metabolic complications
- Both under- and overhydration can be avoided by rigorous fluid balance charts. Do not forget that enteral diets count as approximately 90% fluid, i.e. 1000 ml of feed = 900 ml fluid.
- Hyper- or hypoglycaemia can be caused by inappropriate feeding regimens (*see* overfeeding below) and should be monitored and managed appropriately with the help of a dietitian and insulin/oral hypoglycaemics for diabetic patients.
- Vitamin/trace element deficiencies are rare as most commercially available feeds are now nutritionally complete. Patients receiving small volumes of feed over a prolonged period of time may be at risk. *See* Table 4.6 for details of clinical syndromes. Appropriate monitoring should avoid problems.

Overfeeding
Overfeeding, i.e. giving calories in excess of requirements, can be a significant problem, and there are several metabolic complications associated with it, especially in the critically ill patient. These complications can be very serious and even fatal.

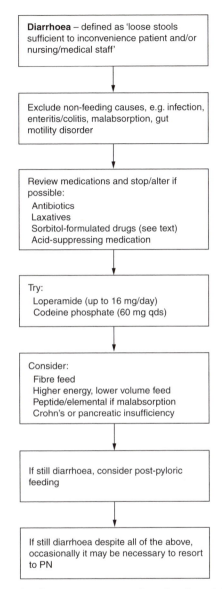

Figure 5.6   Enteral feeding diarrhoea: management algorithm for adults.

- *Hyperglycaemia.* This is especially important in critically ill patients where it has been found that controlling blood glucose levels within 4–6 mmol/l reduces mortality (van den Berghe *et al.*, 2001 – *see* further reading list).
- *Hypercapnoea.* Nutrient metabolism requires oxygen and produces carbon dioxide. Overfeeding should be avoided as greater amounts of CO_2 are produced, and this can delay weaning from a ventilator or cause problems for patients with significant respiratory disease.
- *Azotaemia.* Catabolism and excessive protein intake contribute to this.
- *Hypertonic dehydration.* This can be due to excessive protein intake combined with inability to excrete nitrogenous waste effectively. This occurs with patients who are dehydrated.

Causes of overfeeding include:

- inaccurate nutritional assessment
- not taking into consideration energy from non-feed sources, e.g. propofol, glucose containing dialysate solutions
- basing nutritional requirements on weight without taking into account oedema/ascites (*see* Table 3.1)
- attempting to meet nitrogen losses – catabolic patients can lose as much as 35 g of nitrogen/day – and this cannot be made up with feeding.

To prevent overfeeding:

- careful calculation of nutritional requirements is needed. This should be done by a dietitian or suitably qualified person
- do not attempt to meet nitrogen losses – very catabolic patients cannot achieve positive nitrogen balance
- monitor carefully
- it is safer to underfeed rather than overfeed, especially critically ill patients who are more metabolically unstable.

Refeeding syndrome
- Refeeding syndrome (*see* Figure 5.7) is a term to describe the various metabolic complications that can arise as a result of feeding undernourished patients, e.g. anorexia nervosa.

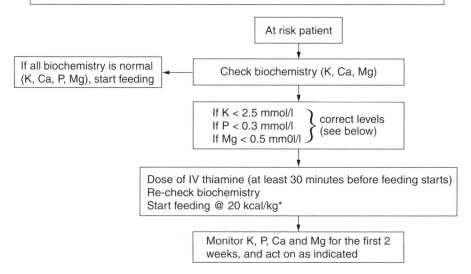

Defined as severe fluid and electrolyte shifts and related metabolic implications in malnourished patients undergoing refeeding. Signs are hypophosphataemia, hypokalaemia, hypomagnesaemia, altered glucose metabolism, fluid balance abnormalities, vitamin deficiency

At risk patient

If all biochemistry is normal (K, Ca, P, Mg), start feeding ← Check biochemistry (K, Ca, Mg)

If K < 2.5 mmol/l
If P < 0.3 mmol/l
If Mg < 0.5 mmol/l } correct levels (see below)

Dose of IV thiamine (at least 30 minutes before feeding starts)
Re-check biochemistry
Start feeding @ 20 kcal/kg*

Monitor K, P, Ca and Mg for the first 2 weeks, and act on as indicated

*20 kcal/kg for the first 24 hrs, then increase gradually within the first week to full feeding, with careful monitoring and replenishing of electrolytes as required. The dietitian will advise on the feeding regimen and rate, but the clinical team has responsibility for correcting fluid and electrolyte imbalances prior to starting enteral feeding.

Figure 5.7 Prevention and management of refeeding syndrome.

- Undernourished patients are catabolic and their major sources of energy are fat and muscle. Serum concentrations of phosphate, magnesium and potassium are kept normal by adjustments in renal excretion. If this catabolic drive is suddenly reversed to anabolism by the administration of excessive carbohydrate, there is a surge of insulin secretion, which causes massive cellular uptake of phosphate, magnesium and potassium and a consequent fall in serum levels. This can cause dangerous arrhythmias and neurological events, and can be fatal.
- In addition, all the problems seen in overfeeding can occur in refeeding (*see* above).

Such patients therefore must *never* be fed over appropriate requirements however emaciated they may be. For example a female weighing 30 kg should not be given more than 600 kcal/day (20 kcal/kg) maximum to start with.

Replacement treatment
- Low phosphate (<0.3 mmol/l):
  - 40 mmol in 500 ml 5% dextrose over 6 hours. Shake bag well
  - oral phosphate causes diarrhoea.
- Low magnesium (<0.5 mmol/l):
  - 6 g (50% $MgSO_4$) in 500 ml 5% dextrose over 6–12 hours
  - oral magnesium is poorly absorbed due to gastrointestinal side-effects of large doses.
- Low potassium (<2.5 mmol):
  - IV fluids containing potassium, e.g. 40 mmol K in 1000 ml N Saline over 8 hours. Repeat as necessary
  - or oral potassium 40–60 mmol/day.
- Thiamine:
  - 200–300 mg IV in 50–100 ml 5% dextrose over 30 minutes.

Further reading

- Bowling TE (1995) Enteral feeding-related diarrhoea: proposed causes and possible solutions. *Proc Nutr Soc.* **54**: 579–90.
- Bowling TE and Silk DBA (1994) Enteral feeding – problems and solutions. *Clin Nutr.* **48**: 379–85.
- Cook MA, Hally V and Panteli JV (2001) The importance of refeeding syndrome. *Nutrition.* **17**: 632–7.
- Drakulovic MB, Torres A, Bauer TT *et al.* (1999) Supine body position as a risk factor for nosocomial pneumonia in mechanically ventilated patients: a randomised trial. *Lancet.* **354**: 1851–8.
- Klein CJ, Stanek GS and Wiles CE (1998) Overfeeding macronutrients to critically ill adults: metabolic complications. *J Am Diet Assoc.* **98**: 795–806.
- McClave SA, DeMeo MT, DeLegge MH *et al.* (2002) North American Summit on Aspiration in the Critically Ill Patient: Consensus Statement. *JPEN.* **26**: S80–5.
- van den Berghe G, Wouters P, Weekers F *et al.* (2001) Intensive insulin therapy in critically ill patients. *N Engl J Med.* **345**: 1359–67.

Parenteral feeding

Definition

Parenteral nutrition (PN) is the administration of nutrient solutions *via* a central or peripheral vein.

Indications

PN is an expensive way to feed patients and has a greater and more serious risk of complications than enteral feeding. Furthermore, it is not more effective than enteral feeding and, therefore, should only be used when the gut is either not working or is inaccessible.

It is important to note that the provision of PN for less than 7 days is unlikely to have any clinical or financial benefit.

A number of trials has demonstrated improved clinical outcome in certain groups, which are accepted indications for PN.

- *Pre-operative feeding.* (*See* Chapter 6 for more details.)
  - Pre-operative feeding of patients with *severe* malnutrition (BMI $< 17 \, \text{kg/m}^2$) undergoing major resectional surgery has been shown to have a decreased incidence of septic complications.
  - Patients less severely malnourished have an increase in non-infectious complications, and therefore should not be fed intravenously.
  - Although inadequately tested in trials, such feeding should be oral/enteral where possible.
  - Pre-operative feeding (enteral or parenteral) is only likely to be effective if given for greater than 10 days.
- *Post-operative feeding.* (*See* Chapter 6 for more details.)
  - PN increases morbidity by 10% and, therefore, should not be used routinely.
  - Well nourished patients undergoing major surgery in whom it is envisaged that they will be unable to be fed enterally for more than 10–14 days. PN should be commenced at about 7 days post-operatively.
  - Patients who are well/adequately nourished at the time of surgery and are still not eating or drinking 7–10 days post-operatively because of complications – although enteral feeding, e.g. by jejunostomy or NJ tube, may be more appropriate (*see* above, routes for enteral feeding).
- Proximal gastrointestinal tract fistulae of whatever aetiology. (Distal fistulae involving colon or rectum can be managed without PN.)
- Patients with multiple organ dysfunction syndrome or following major trauma where nutritional requirements cannot be met *via* the enteral route (*see* p. 92).
- Post-chemotherapy mucositis where passage of an NG tube is contraindicated and where malabsorption may occur throughout the small bowel.

Indications for long-term PN include:

- extensive Crohn's disease unable to support nutrient absorption
- high output fistulae

- short bowel syndrome
- motility disorders: pseudo-obstruction, visceral myopathy/neuropathy
- radiation enteritis.

Details and techniques of long-term (home) PN are beyond the scope of this publication.

Routes

PN should be administered through a dedicated feeding line *via* a volumetric pump suitable for high risk therapies.

The following routes are available for short-term feeding (less than 28 days).

- Central line.
- Peripherally-inserted central catheter (PICC).
- Peripherally-inserted catheter (PIC).
- Peripheral cannula.

Table 5.10   Options for central catheters

Site	Sepsis rates	Mechanical complications	Management problems
Subclavian	Low rate	Moderate complication risk Pneumothorax and thoracic duct injury are highest risks in this area	Shoulder movement if sutured laterally Contamination by tracheal or oral secretions Contraindicated for patients with thrombocytopaenia
Jugular	Higher rate	Moderate complication risk Horner's syndrome, brachial plexus injury and thrombosis are highest risks in this area	Difficult dressing application; neck movement loosens dressing Contamination by hair, tracheal or oral secretions
Femoral	Highest rate	Lower complication risk (except sepsis) Thrombosis and immobility complications are highest risks in this area	Site easily contaminated by urine or faeces Difficult to place and maintain dressing due to movement
Basilar or cephalic (i.e. PICC)	Very low rate	Low complication risk	Easy dressing placement Very low contamination risk

Central line
- *See* Table 5.10 for central catheter options.
- Greater complication rates for insertion.
- Ideally single lumen lines should be used exclusively for PN.
- The exclusive use of one lumen in a multi-lumen line has a greater risk of line sepsis. Practicalities of patient management, especially in the critical care setting, often require multi-lumen lines.
- The major complication is line sepsis. Lines, therefore, need careful handling (*see* below).
- The subclavian route is preferred to the jugular or femoral routes as the latter two have higher infection rates and it is more difficult to maintain sterile dressings.

PICC
- The PICC is inserted into vein in antecubital fossa and about 60 cm in length. The proximal end lies in the central veins thereby allowing hyperosmolar 'central' menus to be tolerated.
- Requires aseptic technique for insertion and should be done by trained personnel.
- Needs good size veins.
- With good care PICCs can last many months and are, therefore, a very good alternative to central lines. Indeed some authorities prefer this route.
- Major complications, other than failure to insert, are phlebitis (5–15%), malposition (8%) and catheter failure/leakage (4%).

PIC
- The PIC is also inserted into mid arm veins, but is only typically 20 cm long. The proximal end, therefore, is in axillary vein and hence only 'peripheral' strength regimens can be given – hyperosmolar 'central' feeds risk causing thrombophlebitis.
- Little published data on efficacy but probably little, if anything, to recommend over PICC.
- Unsuitable for most paediatric patients due to inability to infuse optimal calories.

Peripheral cannula
- Can be used, but its place as a route of first choice is contentious.
- Such lines are easier to insert than a central line, PICC or PIC, and with meticulous care can be maintained for several weeks.
- To optimise efficacy:
  - fine bore (22 or 24 FG polyurethane cannula)
  - large forearm vein
  - hypocaloric, i.e. low osmolality, feed
  - glyceryl trinitrate patch *distal* to cannula
  - regular change of line (at least 48 hourly).
- Unsuitable for most paediatric patients due to inability to infuse optimal calories.

Other considerations
- If peripheral lines are used (i.e. cannulae or PIC) then only low osmolality ('strength') feeds can be administered. If full 'strength' feeds are given thrombophlebitis is likely to result. Therefore, over time, the patient fed peripherally will receive much less nutrition, which may be detrimental. This is *the* major

---

Box 5.1   Recommendation

- Overall, for short-term feeding (<28 days) in the hospital setting, the preferred option would be a PICC or single lumen central catheter. Where venous access is required for multiple purposes, e.g. in the critical care setting, it may be more pragmatic to accept one lumen of a multi-lumen catheter to be exclusively designated to PN. If peripheral cannulae are to be used, meticulous attention must be given to the technique.
- For long-term feeding (>28 days) tunnelled central lines with a dacron cuff (e.g. Hickman or Broviac catheters) or an implantable venous access disc will be required. Details and techniques of long-term (home) PN are beyond the scope of this publication.

---

drawback of peripheral feeding, and will hence be unsuitable for patients with high nutritional requirements.
- Venous integrity and anatomy should be considered and assessed prior to any line insertion. This is particularly relevant for PICC and PIC lines.
- *See* recommendation, Box 5.1.

Practical considerations

Line insertion
Details of line insertion are not given. This needs to be done under strict aseptic conditions by experienced individuals. Local policy/protocol should be adhered to.

Dressings
- After a PICC or PIC line is inserted, a sterile gauze dressing covers the insertion site for the first 24 hours. Thereafter the gauze is removed and a sterile transparent occlusive dressing should cover the insertion site.
- For central lines, use either a sterile gauze or a transparent semi-permeable dressing.
- Dressings should be changed at least weekly, or at any time should the dressing become soiled, wet or loose.
- Dressing change should be done using a strict aseptic technique.

Insertion site
- Insertion site, whatever line/route has been selected, should be inspected daily.
- If there are any signs of inflammation or extravasation, the clinical team or the nutritional support team will need to review the situation and consider appropriate management.

Administering PN
- *See* Table 5.11.
- The prepared feed must not be administered until an X-ray has checked the position of the catheter, unless a peripheral cannula is being used.
- The prepared bag must be stored in a refrigerator and taken out approximately 2 hours prior to use to allow it to warm up to room temperature.

Table 5.11 Administration of PN. (Refer to local policy/protocols if available)

Equipment required

PN bag	Infusion pump	Dressing pack
PN prescription chart	PN administration set	Alcohol spray

Action	Rationale
1 Use strict aseptic technique	To reduce risk of extrinsic infection
2 Wash hands	
3 Check PN bag with prescription and patient in accordance with administration of medicines policy	To ensure patient is receiving correct bag/regimen
4 Open dressing pack and assemble equipment. Place PN container on top of trolley, wipe ports with alcohol and allow to dry	To allow time for antiseptic to work
5 Place sterile clinical sheet below patient's catheter hub, spray with chlorhexidine gluconate or povidone-iodine unless contraindicated by the manufacturer's recommendations	
6 Put on sterile gloves and attach dedicated administration set to PN container and prime set manually	To ensure fluid is free-flowing
7 Attach primed administration set to the patient	
8 Load administration set into pump at calculated rate (see sheet prescription accompanying PN bag)	
9 Ensure the connection is secure and not leaking. Administration set may be taped to patient's arm	To reduce the risk of infection and prevent accidental removal
10 Sign prescription chart and document on fluid balance chart	

Line removal
- Central line removal to be done in accordance with local hospital policy.
- PICC/PIC line removal.
  - Use aseptic technique.
  - Remove occlusive dressing.
  - Gently withdraw catheter.

– Apply pressure to the insertion site to achieve haemostasis.
– Examine line tip. If patient is pyrexial or there are signs of sepsis, line tip should be sent to microbiology for culture.
• Peripheral cannulae can be removed simply by withdrawing and applying pressure until haemostasis has been achieved.

Monitoring

• Regular monitoring of patients receiving PN is essential to ensure safe and effective nutritional therapy.
• Line care must be meticulous. All hospitals should have local protocols for this, and these should be followed.
• Monitoring must include clinical (bedside), nutritional and biochemical parameters.

Tables 5.12, 5.13 and 5.14 are to be used as a guide only and local practice must be followed.

Bedside and nutritional monitoring
This information should be recorded by the nursing staff. *See* Table 5.12.

Biochemical monitoring
• *See* Tables 5.13 and 5.14.
• The frequency of biochemical monitoring should be based on the clinical status of the individual patients. These guidelines should be followed for the majority of patients.
• When patients become stable, the frequency of biochemical testing can decrease.

Complications

Complications of PN can be divided into:

• insertion-related complications
• line-related complications
• feeding-related complications.

Insertion-related complications
Central venous cannulation can lead to the following early complications.

• Failure to insert.
• Pneumothorax.
• Arterial puncture.
• Air embolism.
• Haemothorax.
• Haemopericardium ± cardiac tamponade.
• Arrhythmias.
• Central venous thrombosis.
• Phrenic, vagus or recurrent laryngeal nerve and brachial plexus injury.
• Thoracic duct injury ± chylothorax.

Table 5.12 Bedside and nutritional monitoring of patients receiving PN. (Refer to local policy/protocols if available)

Parameter	Frequency	Notes
Clinical condition of patient	Daily (minimum)	Observe closely for changes, e.g. pyrexia, vomiting, diarrhoea, increased GI losses. Inform clinicians if necessary
Temperature, blood pressure and pulse	Twice daily (minimum)	Pyrexia, tachycardia and hypotension could all be associated with sepsis, e.g. catheter infection. Patient requires urgent review by clinicians or nutrition team
Blood glucose	Every 12 hours for 2 days, then daily (unless patient is diabetic)	Hypo- or hyperglycaemia indicates changes to PN menu may be required. Inform clinicians, dietitians and/or nutrition team
Fluid balance	Daily	Record fluid input/output over 24 hours to indicate fluid overload/ dehydration
Catheter entry site	Daily	Follow local practice when handling catheter Inform clinicians if any problems, e.g. erythema, phlebitis, extravasation
Weight	Daily initially, then twice weekly	Fluid balance Plot on weight chart or centile chart in paediatrics Inform consultant/nutrition team if weight decreases over 2 or more weeks in adults, 2 or more days in infants and children under 2, and 1 week in children 1–10 years
Height	Once only	Useful only for assessing BMI and centile charts in paediatrics Record in notes
Total calorie intake	Daily	Calculate PN administered *versus* PN prescribed. Inform PN pharmacist if less than 90% administered For patients receiving a combination of PN with enteral nutrition or food, ensure an accurate record of intake is maintained and reviewed daily by dietitians or nutrition team

Table 5.13 Biochemical monitoring of patients receiving PN. (Refer to local policy/protocols if available)

Parameter	Initial baseline	Daily	Twice weekly	Weekly	Monthly
Sodium	✓	✓			
Potassium	✓	✓			
Urea	✓	✓			
Creatinine	✓	✓			
Glucose	✓	✓			
Liver function	✓		✓		
Calcium	✓		✓		
Phosphate	✓		✓		
Magnesium	✓		✓		
Full blood count	✓			✓	
Triglycerides				✓	
Zinc				✓	
Copper					✓
Selenium					✓
Manganese					✓

All of these complications need to be managed appropriately, details of which are beyond the scope of this book.

PICC/PIC line or peripheral cannula insertion can lead to the following.

- Failure to insert.
- Malposition.

Line-related complications
The commonest complication for central lines is infection, and for peripheral lines thrombophlebitis and occlusion. These will be dealt with in detail.

Central catheter infection
Exit site infection
Exit site infection is clearly visible on examination as an exudate, frank pus or inflammation (erythema, tenderness and induration) within 2 cm of the skin exit site.

Treatment
Take local wound swab, clean site thoroughly with antiseptic/dressing as per hospital policy and treat with antibiotics, such as flucloxacillin 500 mg qds for 5 days (adult dose).

Tunnel infection (tunnelled lines only)
Tunnel infection is present when there are signs of inflammation along the track of the catheter beyond the exit site.

Table 5.14 Biochemical monitoring and outcomes for patients receiving PN. (Refer to local policy/protocols if available)

Parameter	Frequency	Notes
Sodium	Daily (once stable twice weekly)	Increased sodium: usually dehydration, rarely sodium excess. Often associated with increased urea. Check fluid balance and consider increased fluid input Decreased sodium: usually fluid overload rather than sodium depletion. Check for losses, e.g. fistula, pyrexia. Check fluid balance and consider decreased fluid input
Potassium	Daily (once stable twice weekly)	Increased potassium: consider sample haemolysis, lipaemia or contaminated sample. Renal failure Decreased potassium: Check for increased GI losses. Check for hypomagnesaemia if resistant to treatment
Urea	Daily (once stable twice weekly)	Increased urea: occurs in renal failure, suggestive of dehydration. Consider increasing fluid input Decreased urea: suggestive of fluid overload or poor nutritional status. Consider decreasing fluid input
Creatinine	Daily (once stable twice weekly)	Elevated in renal failure
Glucose	Monitoring strips, e.g. BM: 3–4 daily until stable, then daily Blood: daily (once stable twice weekly)	Elevated glucose: may be due to sepsis or poorly controlled diabetes. Insulin may be required Hypoglycaemia: may occur if PN stopped abruptly. Consider reducing rate of PN over last 1–2 hours
LFTs	Twice weekly	May be elevated as a result of underlying or pre-existing hepatic disease, drug therapy, sepsis, long-term PN, overfeeding Investigate and treat accordingly
(Corrected) calcium	Twice weekly	Increased calcium: occurs in renal failure Decreased calcium: may be result of refeeding syndrome or phosphate supplementation
Phosphate	Twice weekly	Increased phosphate: occurs in renal failure Decreased phosphate: may be a result of refeeding syndrome or existing alcohol abuse
Magnesium	Twice weekly	Increased magnesium: occurs in renal failure Decreased magnesium: may be result of refeeding syndrome or existing alcohol abuse. May get hypomagnesaemia from increased GI losses
Albumin	Twice weekly	Poor marker of nutritional status. An indicator of disease severity Treat appropriately
Full blood count, clotting screen	Weekly	Low haemoglobin may be associated with lack of iron in PN White cell count rises in infection
Triglycerides	Weekly	If elevated review fat intake
Zinc	Fortnightly	Characteristic rash occurs in deficiency, often associated with poor wound healing. Increased loss in fistula/diarrhoea
Trace elements (copper, selenium, manganese)	Monthly	Long term PN patients only Treat appropriately

Treatment
- Take exit site swabs, peripheral and central blood cultures (aseptically).
- If the patient is clinically stable leave line *in situ* and await results of blood cultures.
- For short-term central venous catheters, consider removing catheter and using peripheral access, or replacing central venous catheter in another site after 24 hours of systemic broad spectrum antibiotics if possible.
- For Hickman/Groshong catheters, take exit site swabs, peripheral and central blood cultures (aseptically), commence systemic antibiotics and contact the nutrition team or appropriate clinician for advice.

Catheter sepsis
Catheter-related sepsis is a serious life threatening infection.

Clinical diagnosis
- Pyrexia of 38–39°C (but check for other sources of infection, i.e. sputum, urine and wound).
- Leucocytosis.
- The same positive cultures from a peripheral blood and central blood or catheter tip.
- Complementary evidence: pyrexia and rigors during infusion.

Treatment
Below is a general guide to treatment of catheter sepsis (*see also* Figure 5.8). However, local policies/protocols, where they exist, should be followed.

- Stop PN.
- Take exit site swabs, peripheral blood cultures and central venous catheter blood cultures from feeding lumen (aseptically).
- While awaiting the results of culture the central venous catheter should be locked with heparin (5000 IU/ml). Alternatively it can be removed and a new line inserted at the same site over a guide wire, providing there is no exit site infection.
- If cultures negative, re-use catheter and observe. If signs of sepsis persist, consider alternative sources, e.g. chest, urine etc.
- If cultures are positive, catheter should be locked with vancomycin to fill the luminal dead-space for 12 hours, and (blind) broad spectrum antibiotics started, as agreed by local hospital policy and in discussion with the microbiologists.
- If there is no improvement after the first 48 hours the catheter, whether the original or the guide wire replaced one, must be removed. In addition systemic antibiotics should be continued, the choice and duration of which will be guided by local advice.
- If improvement, use of the catheter for feeding may recommence 48 hours after the subsidence of symptoms and signs, and after negative blood cultures are obtained from the catheter.
- Catheter salvage should not be attempted with *Candida albicans*, *Staphylococcus aureus* and methicillin-resistant *Staph. aureus* (MRSA) infections, as it is unlikely to succeed, and it should be removed.

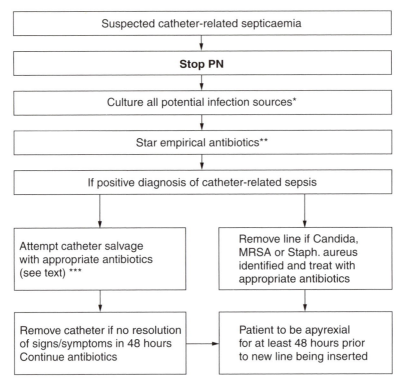

*Including quantitative cultures. Media can be obtained from microbiology.

**Antibiotics should be chosen to cover the likely infecting bacteria,
e.g. vancomycin IV 1 g bd for adults (adjust dose in renal impairment).

***The decision to attempt salvage or remove the line should be based on the
infecting organism, severity of the infection and the availability of alternative
venous access.

Figure 5.8   Algorithm for central catheter-related sepsis (refer to local policy/protocols
if available).

- When a new catheter is required, either because of failed response to antibiotics
  or *Staph. aureus*, MRSA or Candida infection, this must be inserted at an
  alternative site and used only once apyrexial for at least 48 hours.
- If symptom/temperature resolution ± microbiological results are prolonged, the
  patient can be fed peripherally.

Peripheral line infection/thrombophlebitis
If there is any evidence of local discomfort, tenderness, erythema or tracking,
stop the infusion, remove the catheter and send the tip for microbiological culture
and sensitivity. Undertake care of the inflamed site with appropriate cleansing,
dressings and cool packs if required.

Catheter occlusion
Catheter occlusion may be due to kinking, luminal deposition of fibrin, lipid sludge
or amorphous debris. It can affect central catheters, PICC and PIC lines.
   Fibrin occlusion will only occur if blood extravasates into the line. Some central
lines, e.g. Hickman catheters, have a Groshong tip that prevents this happening.

Lipid occlusion only occurs after a more prolonged period of feeding. Therefore early (<7–14 days) occlusion is likely to be due to fibrin, and late (>14 days) is more likely to be due to lipid.

Occasionally medication can cause occlusion. Seek pharmacist advice if this is suspected.

Treatment
Below and in Figure 5.9 is a scheme for managing catheter occlusion. However, local policies, where they exist, should be followed.

- For central catheters, PICC and PIC lines, obtain a chest X-ray in order to check line position.
- Attempt heparinised saline flush (10 units/ml) with 10 ml syringe.
- If still occluded the following methods for unblocking catheters include: 4 ml of 70% ethanol if lipid occlusion is suspected, or urokinase lock (5000 IU in 1 ml for adults, diluted with 2–3 ml normal saline for children) if fibrin occlusion is suspected, with catheter patency attempted after 6 hours.
- It should be noted that urokinase is unlicensed for this use.
  If unsuccessful, lock off lumen, and use another lumen, or change catheter. Never use Y connectors or three-way taps.

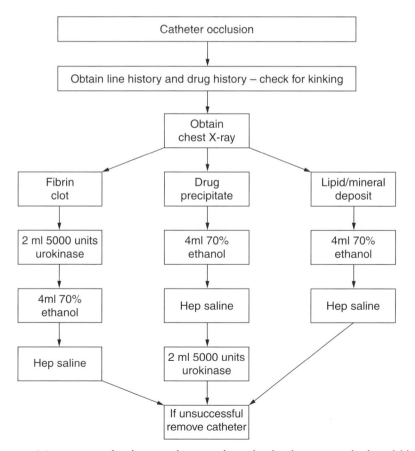

Figure 5.9   Management of catheter occlusion (refer to local policy/protocols if available).

Catheter damage

This can occur when too much force is applied and the catheter splits. It is often as a result of too great a pressure when flushing. Although rare, some lines split when clamps are used on the non-reinforced section of the catheter. Hickman catheters and many PICC/PIC lines can be repaired with an appropriate repair kit provided by the manufacturers. It is vitally important that the line is clamped above the damaged portion to avoid air embolism and infection.

Extravasation

This can occur when the line displaces from the vessel and nutrient solutions then infiltrate surrounding subcutaneous tissue. The line must be removed and the patient must be assessed by the appropriate clinical team to assess for skin damage and to ensure appropriate treament is given straight away.

Feeding-related complications

Metabolic

Deficiencies and excesses of water, electrolytes, vitamins, minerals and trace elements can all happen in patients on PN. Many of the deficiency syndromes only occur after prolonged feeding (>28 days) and are therefore rarely relevant to shorter-term hospital-based PN.

The main problems relevant to short-term feeding (<28 days) relate to fluid balance and glycaemic control.

Appropriate monitoring, as described above, and close communication with the nutrition team (if available) and/or the dietitians and pharmacists should avoid most of these problems.

Hepatobiliary and bone

Cholestasis, cholelithiasis, liver steatosis and cirrhosis can all result from PN, but on the whole are not problems seen in short-term feeding. Further information can be found in the further reading list.

Discontinuing PN

When?

- PN should never be stopped abruptly before alternative methods of feeding have been established, as rebound hypoglycaemia can occur.
- Patients should be started on an enteral or oral diet when thought appropriate by the clinical team and/or nutritional support team. PN should be weaned off or discontinued in those patients who are able to tolerate and absorb oral/ enteral feeding.
- At this point, nursing staff or the patient should maintain accurate food record charts, in addition to the existing fluid balance charts.
- In other instances, e.g. the decision for palliative care, it may be appropriate to withdraw PN. This decision will usually be made by the clinical team/nutrition team in association with the patient and relatives/carers.

How?

- Oral or enteral feeding should be introduced as early as the patient's condition allows, initially slowly and increasing gradually to optimal requirements over 1–2 days.
- Those patients who are able to consume regular amounts of food with an energy content of greater than 1000 kcal/day will generally be able to stop PN without any special precautions. Clinical observation by nursing staff, and 4 hourly BMs will identify the rare patient who has problems after cessation.
- For patients where recommencement of oral/enteral feeding is a slower process, the amount of PN given will need to be tailored to their needs. The dietitians or nutrition team will advise appropriately.
- If PN needs to stop suddenly or unexpectedly, e.g. line problems, an infusion of 10% dextrose should be initiated at 100 ml/hr for 5 hours, to prevent the problems of rebound hypoglycaemia. Beyond this time, or where patients have ongoing large fluid losses or requirements, additional IV fluids and electrolytes should be administered as clinically indicated.

Line removal

- Central lines ought to be removed once PN is stopped, providing they are not required for any other reason.
- PICCs and peripheral short-term devices may be removed at ward level by nursing staff with the appropriate training.

Further reading

- American Gastroenterological Association (2001) AGA technical review on parenteral nutrition. *Gastroenterology.* **121**: 970–1001.
- American Gastroenterological Association (2001) Medical Position Statement: parenteral nutrition. *Gastroenterology.* **121**: 966–9.
- Buchman A (2002) Total parenteral nutrition-associated liver disease. *JPEN.* **26**: S43–8.
- Department of Health (2001) Guidelines for preventing infections associated with the insertion and maintenance of central venous catheters. *J Hosp Inf.* **47** (Suppl): S47–67.
- Duerkse DR, Papineau N, Siemens J *et al.* (1999) Peripherally inserted central catheters for parenteral nutrition: a comparison with centrally inserted catheters. *JPEN.* **23**: 85–9.
- Kohlhardt SR and Smith RC (1989) Fine-bore silicone catheters for peripheral intravenous nutrition in adults. *BMJ.* **229**: 1380–1.
- Maroulis J and Kalfarentzos F (2000) Complications of parenteral nutrition at the end of the century. *Clin Nutr.* **19**: 295–304.
- Seidner DL (2002) Parenteral nutrition-associated metabolic bone disease. *JPEN.* **26**: S37–42.
- Thompson SE (1999) Insertion of peripherally inserted central catheters for the administration of total parenteral nutrition. *Nutr Clin Pract.* **14**: 191–3.

Drug–nutrient interactions

The definition of a drug–nutrient interaction is:

> An event which occurs when a nutrient availability is altered by a medication, or when a drug effect is altered by an adverse reaction caused by the intake of a nutrient or food.
>
> (ASPEN Guidelines 2002)

- Many patients receiving artificial nutrition are also on complex oral and/or parenteral drug regimens so are at risk of developing problems due to drug–nutrient interactions.
- The effects of drug–nutrient interactions can range from a theoretical risk through to a potentially life threatening problem.
- Interaction may cause nutritional deficiencies, adverse drug effects or failure of drug therapy.

Careful and regular review of drug therapy in patients on artificial nutrition is therefore essential.

Factors influencing drug–nutrient interactions

There are many factors which will influence the nature and significance of any interaction that may occur.

- *Patient profile.* Infants, children, the elderly and patients with organ insufficiency are at increased risk of developing interactions.
- *Nutrition regimen.* It is important to identify the type of nutrition whether it is oral supplements (sip feeds), enteral tube feeding or PN. As a general rule drugs should not be added to any type of feed.
- *Type of feeding tube.* It must be established which type of tube is being used and where it is positioned. The method of delivery may also have an effect on the interaction.
- *Flushing.* Flushing before and after giving each drug will reduce the chance of an interaction occurring. It is important to follow local protocols if they exist.
- *Drugs.* Patients on drugs with a narrow therapeutic index are at risk of developing adverse effects due to interactions, e.g. digoxin, phenytoin. Therefore such drugs should be monitored closely.

Types of drug–nutrient interactions

Drug–nutrient interactions can be classified as either pharmacokinetic or pharmacodynamic.

- Pharmacokinetic interactions are where the 'nutrient' may affect drug absorption, distribution, metabolism or excretion.
- Pharmacodynamic interaction relates to the effects of the 'nutrient' on the pharmacological action of the drug.

There are many potential drug–nutrient interactions, and where patients are on medication as well as nutritional support, advice from the pharmacist is essential. The interested reader is referred to the further reading list below.

Further reading

- ASPEN Board of Directors and Clinical Guidelines Task Force (2002) Guidelines for the Use of Parenteral and Enteral Nutrition in Adults and Paediatric Patients. *JPEN.* **26** (Suppl 1): 1SA–138SA.
- Beckwith M, Barton R and Graves C (1997) Guide to drug therapy in patients with enteral feeding tubes: dosage form selection and administration methods. *Hosp Pharmacist.* **32**: 57–64.
- Lourenco R (2001) Enteral feeding: drug/nutrient interaction. *Clin Nutr.* **20**: 187–93.
- Thomson F, Naysmith M and Lindsay A (2000) Managing drug therapy in patients receiving enteral and parenteral nutrition. *Hosp Pharmacist.* **7**: 155–64.
- White R and Ashworth A (2000) How drug therapy can affect, threaten and compromise nutritional status. *J Hum Nutr Dietet.* **13**: 119–29.

CHAPTER 6

Peri-operative nutritional support

Introduction

As long ago as 1936, Studley reported that 'weight loss was the basic indicator of surgical risk' and thus the concept of peri-operative nutritional support having some relevance to surgical outcome was born. More recently appreciation that undernutrition is prevalent in up to 40% of hospital admissions has strengthened the need for guidance as to whom and how surgeons should manage nutrition in and around surgical intervention

Far from an established practice, peri-operative nutritional support remains an infrequently and variably addressed therapy, despite significant data to suggest that when given to the appropriate patients and *via* an appropriate route it can significantly reduce post-operative morbidity (in particular infectious complications) and reduce hospital stay.

Rationale

The rationale for good nutritional management in the surgical patient can be justified by the following.

- *Undernutrition*:
  - ↓ muscle function, including respiratory muscles. This will impair ability to clear secretions and increase risk of chest infections
  - causes immune suppression thereby increasing infectious complications
  - causes increased tiredness and depression/apathy, which lead to decreased mobility and delayed return to normal physical function and consequent increased length of stay
  - as a result of the above three, the costs of care are far greater for the undernourished surgical patient compared to the normally-nourished patient.
- *Gut barrier function*. The gut and in particular the colon is said to contain enough bacteria to kill their human 'host' many times over. What prevents this destructive interaction is the presence of the so-called 'gut barrier'. This barrier allows digestion and absorption of vital nutrients, and the interaction of bacteria with the immune system (in health and disease) without overwhelming it. Insults such as trauma, surgery and haemorrhage lead to a breakdown in the normal gut barrier function. Experimentally this leads to translocation of bacteria

(bacteria crossing from the bowel lumen into the systemic circulation) and activation of the systemic inflammatory cascade leading to sepsis and organ failure. These account for a significant percentage of peri-operative deaths. The exact role and importance of translocation in man is a matter for debate, as is the impact of nutritional status and method of nutritional support. However, there are certainly good animal data that starvation and parenteral feeding can both lead to intestinal atrophy, bacterial overgrowth and a detrimental effect on gut mucosal immune function. All of these factors are important in promoting bacterial translocation.

Indications

As a general principle this is a major area of clinical practice that is still unresolved. Who should be fed, how, for how long and with what?

There are many studies on feeding the peri-operative patient: many small, some larger, some prospectively randomised controlled trials, and many more that have less robust methodology.

What follows is a very brief synopsis of the literature, and our interpretation and suggestions from it (*see* Figure 6.1).

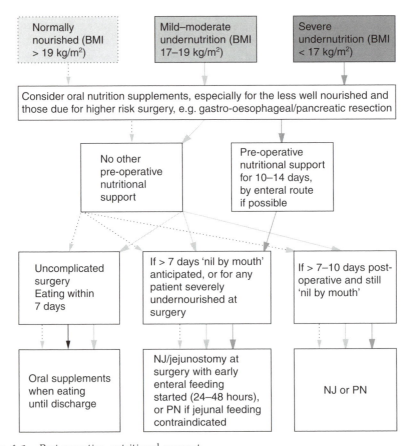

Figure 6.1 Peri-operative nutritional support.

Pre-operative feeding: parenteral/enteral

- Most studies on pre-operative feeding involve PN rather than enteral or oral feeding.
- Patients who are normally nourished or mildly to moderately undernourished do not benefit from pre-operative PN. In fact they have a greater incidence of infectious complications.
- Patients who are severely malnourished, i.e. those with a BMI of $< 17 \, kg/m^2$, do benefit from pre-operative PN, as long as it is given for a minimum of 10 days.
- Most authorities would agree that if enteral feeding is possible this should be the route of choice rather than PN, even though there is no good literature evidence for this.
- Whether it is justifiable to delay surgery for 10+ days to allow nutritional support needs to be considered on an individual basis.
- Ideally nutritional supplementation should be started at the pre-operative clinic/ assessment.

Post-operative feeding: parenteral/enteral

- Normally nourished or mildly undernourished patients do not need any particular nutritional intervention, providing eating has resumed within 7–10 days of surgery.
- Nutritional intervention may be required if the normally nourished or mildly undernourished patient is able only partially to meet nutritional requirements by 10–14 days post-operatively.
- Meta-analysis has shown that PN leads to a 10% increase in post-operative complications, and therefore should not be used unless enteral feeding is contraindicated, i.e. luminal obstruction below the delivery point or enterocutaneous fistulation with high output $> 1000 \, ml/24 \, hrs$, or when the enteral route is not tolerated, e.g. vomiting, severe diarrhoea.
- Oral or enteral feeding should therefore be the route of choice.
- Post-operatively small intestinal motility returns within 12–24 hours, gastric motility within 24–48 hours and colonic motility within 2–3 days. Feeding directly into the small intestine is therefore entirely acceptable within a very short time of surgery. If gastric feeding is undertaken, a pro-motility agent may be required to aid gastric emptying (*see* p. 92 for further details).
- Consideration to the peri-operative placement of a feeding jejunostomy/NJ tube should be made:
  - where a patient is moderately to severely undernourished (BMI $< 17 \, kg/m^2$) at the time of surgery
  - where a patient was fed pre-operatively because of severe undernutrition and who will not feed immediately post-operatively
  - for patients less severely undernourished (BMI $> 17 \, kg/m^2$), where it may be reasonably felt that resumption of eating is likely to be delayed beyond 7 days.
- *See* Table 6.1 for a comparison of enteral and parenteral feeding in the peri-operative patient.

Table 6.1 Comparison of enteral and parenteral feeding in the peri-operative patient

Enteral feeding	Parenteral feeding
Preserves gut barrier function	Probably impairs gut barrier function (in humans)
Less risk of significant clinical complications	Greater risk of significant clinical complications
Does not affect immune response	Can be immunosuppressive

Peri-operative oral nutritional supplements

There is a growing number of studies looking at the use of oral nutritional supplements both pre- and post-operatively.

There are two broad categories: one of standard feeds and one of so-called immune-enhancing diets – IEDs (*see* Chapter 5 for further details, p. 32).

IEDs are feeds with a standard nutritional base but with additions, such as glutamine, ω-3 fatty acids, nucleotides and arginine. The rationale is that their immune-modulating capacity may influence gut barrier function and other aspects of the immune system.

Evidence to date indicates that:

- standard feeds given both pre-admission, pre-operatively as an in-patient, and post-operatively cut down on minor complications and lessen the degree of weight loss
- there is no demonstrable benefit in continuing standard supplements after discharge from hospital
- IEDs given for 5 days pre-operatively (and also post-operatively *via* enteral feeding tube) lessen infectious complications in patients undergoing high risk surgery, such as oesophageal or pancreatic resection
- whether IEDs are superior to standard feeds is still open to debate, as study design, patient groups and dietary regimens differ very considerably between the relatively small number of studies that have directly compared them
- overall, though, the cost of supplements is relatively low, and patients undergoing moderate to major surgical intervention should probably be offered them throughout the peri-operative period.

Popular myths

- Additional nutritional support should not preclude establishing normal diet.
- It is not necessary to await bowel sounds or passage of flatus prior to allowing oral fluid or nutrition. This is because the return of colonic motility takes 2–3 days typically, whereas gastric and small intestinal motility returns much earlier (*see* above).
- Enteral feeding *via* a gastric or jejunal tube may commence early in the post-operative period, i.e. within 24 hours.

- Down stream anastomosis does not preclude commencing enteral feeding in the early post-operative period.
- A rapid fall in serum albumin from near normal pre-operatively to very low within a few days of surgery does not indicate undernutrition. It indicates fluid overload and the post-operative state.

Further reading

- Allison SP and Kinney JM (2000) Perioperative nutrition. *Curr Opin Clin Nutr Metab Care.* **3**: 1–3.
- Bengmark S (1998) Progress in perioperative enteral tube feeding. *Clin Nutr.* **17**: 145–52.
- Bozzetti F (2002) Perioperative nutrition of patients with gastrointestinal cancer. *Br J Surg.* **89**: 1201–2.
- Chung A (2002) Perioperative nutrition support. *Nutrition.* **18**: 207–8.
- Lewis SJ, Egger M, Sylvester PA *et al.* (2001) Early enteral feeding versus 'nil by mouth' after gastrointestinal surgery: systematic review and meta-analysis of controlled trials. *BMJ.* **323**: 773–6.
- Maxfield D, Geehan D and Van Way CW (2001) Perioperative nutritional support. *Nutr Clin Pract.* **16**: 69–73.
- Sax HC (2001) Effect of immune enhancing formulas (IEF) in general surgery patients. *JPEN.* **25**: S19–23.
- Silk DBA and Green CJ (1998) Perioperative nutrition: parenteral *versus* enteral. *Curr Opin Clin Metab Care.* **1**: 21–7.
- Zapas JL, Karakozis S and Kirkpatrick JR (1998) Prophylactic jejunostomy: a reappraisal. *Surgery.* **124**: 715–20.

CHAPTER 7

Nutritional support in disease-specific situations

Acute pancreatitis

Nutritional support in mild to moderate pancreatitis

- There is no evidence that either enteral or parenteral nutrition has a beneficial effect on clinical outcome in mild to moderate acute pancreatitis.
- Assuming normal or near-normal nutritional status at time of presentation, there is no requirement for nutritional support to be instituted in the first 7 days.
- Nutritional therapy needs to be considered earlier if there is pre-existing malnutrition, e.g. acute on chronic pancreatitis.
- Days 1–5:
  - fasting
  - treat cause of pancreatitis
  - analgesics
  - IV fluids and electrolytes.
- Days 3–7:
  - assuming clinical recovery introduce carbohydrate-rich, moderate protein and fat-poor diet
  - resume normal diet by day 7.
- If normal diet is not possible after day 7 because of complications or clinical deterioration, manage as per 'severe' pancreatitis (*see* below).

Nutritional support in severe acute pancreatitis

- Early feeding decreases incidence of nosocomial infections, systemic inflammatory response syndrome (SIRS) and overall disease severity. There is no evidence to support the need for 'gut rest'.
- Nutritional support is therefore essential in severe acute pancreatitis and should be started within the first 24–48 hours.
- Enteral feeding should be attempted in all patients, and this needs to be administered distal to the ampulla of Vater. The route of choice, therefore, is an NJ tube. Parenteral feeding can be used alongside enteral feeding as a supplement when it is not possible to meet requirements enterally.

- Parenteral feeding should only be used exclusively if the patient is unable to tolerate enteral feeding or if it is contraindicated, e.g. paralytic ileus, or if an NJ tube cannot be placed.
- Requirements:
  - energy: 30–35 kcal/kg body weight/day
  - protein: 1.2–1.5 g/kg body weight/day
  - carbohydrates: 3–6 g/kg body weight/day. Keep blood glucose < 10 mmol/l
  - lipids: up to 2 g/kg body weight/day. Keep triglycerides < 12 mmol/l.

Further reading

- Eckerwall G and Andersson R (2001) Review article: early enteral nutrition in severe acute pancreatitis. *Scand J Gastroenterol.* **5**: 449–58.
- Meiier R, Beglinger C, Layer P *et al.* (2002) ESPEN guidelines on nutrition in acute pancreatitis. *Clin Nutr.* **21**: 173–83.

Nutritional support in the critically ill patient
Metabolic response to trauma/critical illness

- A rudimentary understanding of the metabolic response to trauma/critical illness is very useful when it comes to considering nutrition and nutritional support in critically ill patients. (For more details *see* further reading list at the end of this section.)
- There are two metabolic 'phases' following an acute insult, such as trauma.
  - *'Ebb' phase.* Variable duration, often 24–48 hours. Body goes into shock and effectively shuts down, with low cardiac outflow, hypotension and poor tissue/organ perfusion. Also most cell function is depressed. Main clinical priority is resuscitation.
  - *'Flow' phase.* Characterised by the release of catecholamines, glucagons and cortisol (catabolic hormones) as well as insulin (anabolic). To a certain extent the effects of insulin are counteracted by the others and this leads to insulin resistance with consequent hyperglycaemia. This in turn increases risk of sepsis and inflammatory response, both of which further increase the catabolic state. One purpose of the catabolic hormones is to mobilise glucose, fat and amino acids for utilisation from their respective stores.

Nutritional requirements

The goals of nutritional support in the care of the critically ill patient are:

- to minimise negative energy and protein balance and muscle loss by avoiding starvation
- to maintain tissue function, particularly of the immune system and skeletal and respiratory muscle
- to influence beneficially the subsequent period of recovery.

Energy

- The provision of exogenous nutrients is essential to supply the body with appropriate energy substrates to deal with the various metabolic demands and to minimise depletion of body stores.
- Energy requirements rarely exceed 35 kcal/kg/day.
- Overfeeding (provision of excess calories) can lead to a further elevation in energy expenditure – known as the thermic effect of nutrition – and this puts further stress on the various metabolic processes and is therefore detrimental. Energy supply needs to match metabolic demand as closely as possible.

Glucose

- Glucose is the universal energy substrate and can be utilised by nearly all cells. It can also be metabolised anaerobically and therefore is the energy source in hypoxic tissues.
- Glucose is generated from the breakdown of protein (gluconeogenesis), glycogen (glycogenolysis) and glycerol (from lipolysis of fat). Glycogen stores (mainly from the liver) last <24 hours in critical illness, and therefore the predominant source of glucose is from amino acids and glycerol.
- Glucose tolerance is decreased in critical illness because of increased insulin resistance and incomplete glucose oxidation (i.e. utilisation) by injured organs (e.g. liver, muscle, kidney).
- Glucose provision by means of nutritional support ideally needs to be sufficient to minimise the catabolic processes but not to exceed the body's oxidation capacity. If this capacity is exceeded, lipogenesis is enhanced which leads to fatty acid deposition in the liver and other organs, and more CO_2 is generated which can lead to ventilatory problems.
- Glucose calories should constitute 30–70% of total energy intake.

Fat

- Fatty acids are a primary energy substrate in the liver, heart and skeletal muscle. Their oxidation leads to greater calorie provision than an equivalent amount of glucose (9 kcal/g *versus* 4 kcal/g).
- Free fatty acids (and glycerol) come from the breakdown (lipolysis) of fat stores mainly in adipose tissue.
- Fat calories should constitute 15–30% of total energy.

Protein

- Protein breakdown is often dramatic in critical illness. Certain amino acids are oxidised preferentially – branched chain amino acids (valine, leucine and isoleucine) and glutamine – and hence become particularly depleted.
- Protein provision should constitute 15–20% of total energy, at a level of 0.8–2.0 g/kg/day.

Other considerations

- Nutritional assessment needs to be based on clinical and biochemical parameters rather than on functional, anthropometric or immunologic markers as no single indicator is consistent in the critically ill patient.

- Provision of nutritional support should take into account specific organ failures.
- Non-feed sources of calories should also be taken into account, e.g. dextrose (1000 ml 5% dextrose provides 200 kcal), propofol (approximately 1 kcal/ml) and dialysis fluids.
- Hypoalbuminaemia is common in the critically ill − albumin synthesis is reduced secondary to the increased synthesis of acute phase proteins, and is of minimal significance clinically. A low albumin with a raised C-reactive protein (CRP) is indicative of the acute phase response, while a low albumin with a normal CRP is indicative of protein depletion.
- Because of insulin resistance and hyperglycaemia, it is essential to keep blood sugar levels tightly controlled with insulin therapy (van den Berghe *et al.*, 2001).
- Enteral feed delivery can be poor as a consequence of large NG aspirates (*see* below), tube displacement, procedures, diagnostic tests, nursing care/physiotherapy and gastrointestinal complications of enteral feeding such as vomiting.

Choice of feeding route

- Anorexia, nausea, sedation and analgesia, tracheal intubation and impaired consciousness mean intensive care unit (ICU) patients are usually unable to take oral diet.
- Enteral nutrition is the preferred route of nutrient administration − this requires a functioning gut and a relatively haemodynamically stable patient.
- Early enteral feeding (within the first 24 hours of admission to ICU) reduces subsequent mortality and morbidity.
- PN should be considered only where there is a non-functioning gut and should, where possible, be administered *via* a dedicated line. Occasionally it may be required to supplement enteral feeding that may be providing insufficient calories.

Gastric emptying and bowel sounds

- Anaesthesia, sedation and muscle relaxants can all reduce small bowel motility. Absence of bowel sound is not necessarily an indication of ileus and should not prevent a trial of enteral feeding.
- Gastric emptying rates vary throughout the day, with opiates and hyperosmolar or high fat feeds.
- Gastric stasis is a very common phenomenon in the intensive care setting (*see* Box 7.1). In such situations, intragastric feeding can lead to aspiration and

---

Box 7.1 Causes of gastric stasis

- Multiple trauma, head injury.
- Ventilation.
- Post-operative state.
- Intra-abdominal sepsis.
- Diabetic gastroparesis.
- Hypothyroidism.

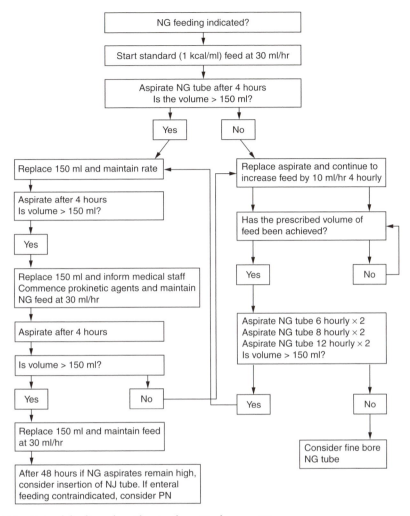

Figure 7.1   Enteral feeding algorithm in the critical care setting.

chest infections. Therefore action is required when there is significant gastric stasis (*see* Figure 7.1).

- Gastric stasis can be managed with regular administration of prokinetic agents such as metoclopramide (10 mg IV tds) or erythromycin (125 mg qds IV), although evidence for efficacy is weak.
- Where gastric feeding still cannot be established, consider post-pyloric feeding (*see* p. 61).

Drug–nutrient interactions

- Bioavailability of certain medicines may be reduced with concurrent enteral feeding, e.g. phenytoin, ciprofloxacin. Seek advice from a pharmacist, monitor therapeutic levels and adjust dose/consider IV preparations if necessary. *See* p. 81 for further details.

Solutions for nutritional support

- At present, standard diets (enteral and parenteral) are adequate for the nutritional support of the critically ill patient.
- Nutritional pharmacology and development of new feeding solutions are rapidly evolving areas, where the aim is to influence morbidity and mortality by providing certain nutrients that can act as pharmacological agents and influence immune function. The following 'novel substrates' are all attracting a great deal of attention.
  - Glutamine has many important functions as a metabolic substrate. Levels drop dramatically in trauma/critical illness.
  - ω-3 polyunsaturated fatty acids inhibit the pro-inflammatory response, unlike ω-6 fatty acids, such as linoleic acid, which stimulate it. Diets are available substituting, in part, ω-6 for ω-3 fatty acids.
  - Arginine stimulates the metabolic response to stress and is a precursor of nitric oxide, a free radical scavenger. Excess or deficiency could be detrimental to patient outcome.
  - Medium chain triglycerides (MCTs) are not precursors of prostaglandin synthesis, unlike long chain triglycerides (LCTs), and hence do not influence the inflammatory/immune response. Diets are available that substitute in part the LCT for MCTs.
  - There are diets which combine a number of 'novel substrates' together, and these have been termed 'immune-enhancing diets' (IEDs).
- Current evidence suggests that use of IEDs is beneficial in (severe) trauma patients, and possibly severe head injury and burn patients. However, overall, despite the wealth of studies and the number of meta-analyses/reviews examining the various 'novel substrate' diets, there is still insufficient evidence to make definitive recommendations regarding their use and advantage over standard diets (enteral or parenteral) in the critical care setting.

Further reading

- Bessey PQ (1996) Metabolic response to trauma and infection. In: JE Fischer (ed) *Nutrition and Metabolism in the Surgical Patient*. Little Brown and Company, Boston, US, pp. 577–601.
- Cerra FB, Benitez MR, Blackburn GL *et al*. (1997) Applied nutrition in ICU patients. A consensus statement of the American College of Chest Physicians. *Chest*. **111**: 769–78.
- Consensus recommendations from the US summit on immune-enhancing enteral therapy (2001) *JPEN*. **25** (Suppl 2): S36–S42.
- Heyland DK, Novak F, Drover JW *et al*. (2001) Should immunonutrition become routine in critically ill patients? A systematic review of the evidence. *JAMA*. **286**: 944–53.
- Mallampalli M, McClave SA and Snider HL (2000) Defining tolerance to enteral feeding in the intensive care unit. *Clin Nutr*. **19**: 213–15.
- Marik PE and Zaloga GP (2001) Early enteral nutrition in acutely ill patients: a systematic review. *Crit Care Med*. **29**: 2264–70.

- McClave SA, Sexton LK, Spain DA *et al.* (1999) Enteral tube feeding in the intensive care unit: factors impeding adequate delivery. *Intensive Care Med.* **27**: 1252–6.
- Montejo JC, Zarazaga A, Lopez-Martinez J *et al.* (2003) Immunonutrition in the intensive care unit. A systematic review and consensus statement. *Clin Nutr.* **22**: 221–33.
- Raper S and Maynard N (1992) Feeding the critically ill patient. *Br J Nurs.* **1**: 273–80.
- Sargent C, Murphy D and Shelton BK (2002) Nutrition in critical care. *Clin J Oncol Nurs.* **6**: 287–9.
- van den Berghe G, Wouters P, Weekers F *et al.* (2001) Intensive insulin therapy in critically ill patients. *N Engl J Med.* **345**: 1359–67.

Nutrition in burn injury

Introduction

The post-burn period is associated with a hypermetabolic state that will result in significant weight loss, delayed wound healing and impaired immune function if nutritional support is not provided. (*See* nutritional support in the critically ill patient, pp. 92–6, for details of the metabolic response to injury.)

Early aggressive nutritional support has been shown to improve survival in burns victims. Mortality and morbidity have also reduced over recent years as a consequence of improvements in fluid and electrolyte management, early excision and skin grafting, the development of artificial and cultured skin, advances in burns dressings and improvements in the management of infections. Multidisciplinary teamwork is vital for the successful treatment of burns patients.

It is important to note that the treatment of burns patients will take place over several weeks or months and that the nutritional requirements of a patient should be regularly reassessed over this time. Feeding regimens should be adjusted to reflect changes in the overall clinical condition. Nutritional therapy as a consequence is complex and requirements should be calculated by a specialist burns dietitian who will not only take into account increased need for protein and energy, but also the altered requirements for vitamins and minerals that occur as a consequence of skin loss, muscle breakdown and increased urinary excretion.

Assessing nutritional requirements

- Predictive equations provide only an estimation of nutritional requirements and do not take into account burn depth or donor sites. Each patient's clinical condition must be considered and monitored regularly.
- Energy requirements for adult burns patients should be assessed using the methodology described in Chapter 4. As a rough guide, for every 1% full thickness burn there is a 1% rise in the stress factor up to a maximum of 50%.
- The estimated requirements may be difficult to achieve, especially in those patients having frequent visits to theatre and those spending prolonged periods of time nil by mouth. The minimum period of fasting necessary peri-operatively

should be agreed with medical and anaesthetic staff. This should then be considered when planning any feeding regimen.

- *Protein* requirements are approximately 20% of total energy, or 1.3–1.5 g protein/ kg/day. Higher levels do not improve nitrogen balance any further.
- *Fluid* requirements should be assessed and monitored daily taking into account the volume supplied by enteral feeding.
- Burns patients may have large losses of *electrolytes* through exudate and increased urinary output. In addition there may be further losses secondary to pyrexia, diarrhoea and/or vomiting. It may be necessary to provide additional sodium and potassium as oral supplements.
- *Micronutrient requirements* of the burns patient will be increased due to their roles in metabolic pathways. Requirements are likely to exceed the dietary reference value (*see* Table 4.6) for patients with >15% body surface area (BSA) burn due to tissue damage, increased muscle breakdown, exudate and increased urinary losses.
- Vitamins and minerals should be prescribed on an individual basis, taking into consideration the amounts supplied by diet, sip and tube feeds. Although there are no specific recommendations for replacement in burns patients, the following points should be considered.
  - Vitamin C has a known role in collagen synthesis. Recommendations suggest total daily intakes of 300–1000 mg/day.
  - High energy intakes, either enterally or parenterally, lead to proportionally increased demands for B Group vitamins.
  - Vitamin A deficiency may play a role in causing stress ulcers due to thinning of the gut epithelium.
- Burns patients may be at risk of *trace element deficiency*, e.g. copper and selenium, because of:
  - increased requirements
  - increased losses – *via* plasma exudate, removal of eschar, urinary and blood losses, diarrhoea and vomiting
  - reduced intake – time spent nil by mouth, inadequate supplementation
  - malnutrition on admission – particularly the elderly, those in institutional care, drug or alcohol abusers.

Trace elements are required for immune function, as co-factors in enzyme systems, as antioxidants, and for wound healing. They are all vital in burn recovery. The use of trace element preparations may be indicated where there is inadequate intake via sip and enteral tube feeds.

When to start feeding

- Patients with *minor burns* (i.e. <10–15% BSA burn in adults) should be encouraged to start eating and drinking from admission. Milk based fluids/sip feeds should be offered in preference to water, squash, pop etc.
- It is recommended that all *shock burn* patients (i.e. >15% BSA burn in adults) are fed *within 6 hours* of admission. Ideally the feeding tube should be placed during the resuscitation period as this is when the majority of invasive treatment occurs.

Feeding route

- Oral feeding is the route of choice for minor burns.
- NG feeding is the preferred option where eating/drinking is either not possible, e.g. facial injury, or not feasible. This is because burns, in contrast to other types of major trauma, have little effect on gastric emptying.
- Patients with BSA burns >20% are likely to require tube feeding, even if they are able to eat and drink, as their requirements are liable to exceed their capacity for oral intake.
- In those situations where there is delayed gastric emptying, post-pyloric enteral feeding should be started.
- Parenteral feeding should be avoided wherever possible because of the increased risk of sepsis.

Patient monitoring

No single parameter is an adequate marker of nutritional status in the short term, but the following measurements are all of relevance and should be repeated regularly.

- *Weight.* Weight should be measured at least weekly without dressings or prior to dressing changes (dressings can subsequently be removed and weighed).
- *Daily food and fluid intake charts.*
- *Nitrogen balance.* Ideally to be measured daily for the first 2 weeks for all shock cases as a measure of catabolism and imminent sepsis (see p. 20 for details). Thereafter, 24 hour urine collections should be made over 2 consecutive days each week.
- *Biochemistry and haematology* (*see* Table 7.1).
- *Clinical condition.* It is important to consider infections, ventilation and other factors likely to influence the patient's metabolic rate and thus energy requirements.

Table 7.1   Monitoring for the burns patient

Parameter	Frequency of measurement
Serum albumin	Twice weekly
CRP	Twice weekly
Serum glucose	Daily for first week
Urea and electrolytes	Daily for first week
LFTs	Twice weekly
Serum calcium and phosphate	Phosphate daily for first week, then weekly. Corrected calcium weekly
Serum copper, zinc, magnesium	Days 7, 14, 21 for BSA burn >20%
Haemoglobin, WCC	Twice weekly for first month (minimum)

- *Hyperglycaemia.* Burns patients may become insulin resistant as part of the metabolic response to trauma, resulting in temporary hyperglycaemia and the need for insulin.
- *BSA burn.* This should be reassessed by experienced medical and nursing staff at each dressing change. As the burn size changes so nutritional requirements will also alter. However, grafted areas should not be treated as healed areas for the first month. NB: donor sites will contribute to the area left to heal.
- *Bowel action.*
- *Temperature.*

Discharge protocol

- Patients who have been receiving a high level of nutritional support should be encouraged to reduce their intake to normal prior to discharge, i.e. equivalent to the estimated average requirement for energy and the reference nutrient intake for other nutrients.
- Those patients who have not achieved their target weight at discharge should be followed up as out-patients by the dietitian as required.

Further reading

- Dickerson RN (2002) Estimating energy and protein requirements of thermally injured patients: art or science? *Nutrition.* **18**: 439–42.
- Gosling P and Hubbard LD (1995) Serum copper and zinc concentrations in patients with burns in relation to BSA. *J Burn Care Rehabilitation.* **16**: 481–6.
- Gottschlich MM and Warden GD (1990) Vitamin supplementation in the patient with burns. *J Burn Care Rehabilitation.* **11**: 275–9.
- Matsuda T, Kagan RJ, Hanumadass M *et al.* (1983) The importance of burn wound size in determining the optimal calorie:nitrogen ratio. *Surgery.* **94**: 562–8.
- Nelson JL (1992) Metabolic and immune effects of enteral ascorbic acid after burn trauma. *Burns.* **8**: 92–7.
- Williams GJ and Herndon DN (2002) Modulating the hypermetabolic response to burn injuries. *J Wound Care.* **11**: 87–9.

Renal disease

- Nutritional therapy is key in the management of patients with renal disease. The main aims of nutritional intervention are:
  - to minimise uraemic toxicity
  - prevent undernutrition.
- Undernutrition is common in renal disease affecting >40% of patients beginning renal replacement therapy. It is associated with poor clinical outcome and mortality and earlier requirement for renal replacement therapy.
- Causes of undernutrition are multifactorial, and include:
  - poor dietary intake exacerbated by dialysis and gastrointestinal symptoms of uraemia, such as nausea, anorexia and diarrhoea
  - metabolic acidosis, which increases protein breakdown
  - ↑ catabolism.

Table 7.2 Nutritional management of renal disease. (Adapted from Hartley and Roberts, 2001)

	Protein	Energy	Potassium	Phosphate	Sodium and fluid
Clinical significance	Need sufficient to avoid malnutrition. Protein restriction is controversial in CRF (*see* text)	Need adequate energy intake to prevent/correct undernutrition	Hyperkalaemia may cause cardiac arrhythmias/cardiac arrest	Hyperphosphataemia contributes to the development of renal bone disease	Excess intake results in fluid overload and hypertension
CRF					
Conservative management	0.8–1.0 g/kg body weight	35 kcal/kg body weight	Restrict if hyperkalaemic	Restriction to 30 mmol/day usually required	No added salt (NAS) if hypertensive. NAS and fluid restriction if overloaded
Haemodialysis	1.0–1.2 g/kg ideal body weight (IBW)	≥35 kcal/kg IBW	Restriction usually required to 1 mmol/kg body weight	Restriction to 30 mmol/day usually required	NAS and fluid restriction usually required
CAPD	>1.2 g/kg IBW	>35 kcal/kg IBW (including glucose absorbed from dialysate)	Restrict if hyperkalaemic. Supplement if hypokalaemic	Restriction to 30–40 mmol/day usually required	NAS and fluid restriction usually required
ARF	≥1 g/kg body weight	Matched to requirements	As required	As required	As required

- It is important to tailor nutritional requirements to the patient's clinical condition, treatment and blood biochemistry. As a guide, refer to Table 7.2.
- Nutritional assessment (*see* Chapter 3) should take into account the presence of oedema and calculations should be based on ideal or usual, rather than actual, body weight.

Chronic renal failure

- The nutritional requirements for patients pre-dialysis and on dialysis are outlined in Table 7.2.

Conservative treatment
- Protein restrictions in the conservative management of chronic renal failure (CRF) patients remain controversial and may in fact contribute to protein–energy malnutrition.
- Energy requirements are high (35 kcal/kg/day) and patients may need oral supplements to achieve adequate intake.

Other considerations.

- Hypertension should be managed to delay the rate of progression of CRF.
- Anaemia is a common complication of CRF – usually treated with recombinant human erythropoeitin and if successfully managed will improve quality of life and cardiovascular stability, and may delay the need for renal replacement therapy.
- Renal bone disease (renal osteodystrophy) occurs as a consequence of hyperphosphataemia and hypocalcaemia. Phosphate should be controlled by dietary restriction ± phosphate binders and hypocalcaemia corrected with activated vitamin D or a vitamin D analogue, e.g. alphacalcidol.

Haemodialysis
- Haemodialysis is a catabolic process with 10–13 g of amino acids lost per day in the dialysate. Therefore protein must be supplied at levels of 1.0–1.2 g/kg/day (*see* Table 7.2).
- It is important to try and optimise nutritional status prior to starting dialysis as deficiencies are more difficult to correct once dialysis has started.
- Fluid restrictions may mean that it is difficult to meet protein and energy requirements.

Chronic ambulatory peritoneal dialysis
- Approximately 50% of chronic ambulatory peritoneal dialysis (CAPD) patients are malnourished – firstly due to heavy protein losses across the peritoneum during the dialysis dwell time, and secondly due to reduced food intake because of satiety and fullness arising from the presence of the infused dialysate fluid in the peritoneal cavity. As with haemodialysis, it is important to try and optimise nutritional status prior to starting dialysis as deficiencies are more difficult to correct once it has started.
- Protein intake should be adequate to compensate for dialysate losses of 5–15 g/day, and normally would be 1.2–1.5 g/kg/day. These losses will increase in the

presence of peritonitis, and an extra 0.1–0.2 g/kg/day should be provided in this situation.
- Approximately 300 kcal/day will be gained by the patient by absorption of glucose from the dialysate fluid – this amount will increase with the use of more hypertonic bags. This should be taken into consideration when calculating feeding regimens.
- Nutritional requirements are outlined in Table 7.2.
- Additional supplementation of thiamin, pyridoxine and vitamin C may be required.

Acute renal failure

- The aim of treatment is to maintain nutritional status and limit the complications of acute renal failure (ARF). Management will be complicated by variations in the disease state, the type of renal replacement therapy and altered metabolism.
- *Non-catabolic ARF.* Normal protein and energy requirements should be met, and fluid and electrolytes should be given according to blood biochemistry and fluid balance. These patients can usually meet their nutritional requirements from normal diet ± nutritional supplements (1.2–1.5 kcal/ml energy density).
- *Catabolic ARF.* This group of patients will often have multi-organ failure and be managed on ICU, and their protein, energy, fluid and other nutritional requirements will be determined by the overall clinical situation, of which ARF is only part (*see* nutritional support in the critically ill patient, pp. 92–6).
- Even if not ventilated, such catabolic patients are unlikely to have an adequate oral intake, even with dietary supplements. NG or NJ tube feeding is often required. IV feeding will be needed if there are significant gastrointestinal tract symptoms, such as vomiting, diarrhoea or ileus.
- The chosen method of renal replacement therapy will also influence the feeding regimen. An appropriately experienced dietitian will need to advise.
- The clinical condition of patients with ARF can change rapidly and close monitoring is essential, e.g. to prevent fluid overload where a urine output decreases or the type of renal replacement therapy changes.

Solutions for nutritional support

- Where tube feeding is required, a standard polymeric diet is usually adequate. 1.5–2.0 kcal/ml feeds may be useful in managing patients on fluid restrictions.
- Specialised 'renal' feeds with low modified protein, potassium and phosphate content are available and may be used where clinically indicated.
- If IV feeding is required, standard solutions are adequate. PN bags may need to be low volume and low electrolyte/electrolyte free based on the overall clinical condition of the patient.

Further reading

- Hartley G and Roberts R (2001) Renal disease. In: B Thomas (ed) *Manual of Dietetic Practice* (3e). Blackwell Science, Oxford.

- Toigo G, Aparicio M, Attman PO *et al.* (2000) Expert working group report on nutrition in adult patients with renal insufficiency (part 1 of 2). *Clin Nutr.* **19**: 197–207.
- Toigo G, Aparicio M, Attman PO *et al.* (2000) Expert working group report on nutrition in adult patients with renal insufficiency (part 2 of 2). *Clin Nutr.* **19**: 281–91.

Diabetes mellitus
Considerations

- The most important aim of patient management is to avoid the extremes of hyper- or hypoglycaemia (*see* below).
- Overall the indications and methods of nutritional support and the estimations for energy, protein and lipid requirements are similar to those for non-diabetics with comparable medical problems.
- The stress response to illness and injury is, in itself, diabetogenic and causes insulin resistance. Hence insulin is often required during acute illness in the Type 2 (non-insulin dependent) diabetic, and increased doses of insulin required for the Type 1 (insulin dependent) diabetic. As a result very close monitoring of blood sugar levels is essential.
- Patients with diabetes receiving nutritional support are likely to require an increase in their diabetes medication.
- Type 2 diabetics receiving enteral feeding can stay on their oral hypoglycaemic agents (OHAs), but with a low threshold for starting insulin if sugar levels are unstable. Crushed tablets can be administered *via* the feeding tube or check with pharmacy regarding liquid preparations.
- If possible, stabilise blood glucose levels prior to initiating nutritional support.
- Unstable patients (post-operatively, critically ill) are best managed on sliding scale insulin regimens. Once stable, swap to subcutaneous (SC) injections.
- The dose, timing and type of insulin will depend largely on the type of feeding.
- Where possible, liaise with the diabetes team.

Enteral nutrition

- Enteral feeds produce a more rapid rise in blood glucose levels than the equivalent intake from food – this effect may be exaggerated with bolus feeding rather than continuous feeding using a pump.
- Blood glucose levels should be monitored closely where changes are made to the feeding regimen or where the feed stops unexpectedly. Give IV dextrose if necessary.
- A change to treatment may be necessary where:
  - feed timing or rate changes
  - delivery method of the feed changes, e.g. pump to bolus
  - feed prescription changes – giving more or less carbohydrate
  - poor feed tolerance/vomiting.
- Patients with gastroparesis may require post-pyloric feeding (*see* p. 61).

Diets where a proportion of carbohydrate has been replaced by mono-unsaturated fat have been suggested to improve blood glucose control and lipid profile. These modified carbohydrate feeds, e.g. Glucerna SR (Abbott), Diason (Nutricia), are currently not available in the UK and some other countries. Clinical trials are ongoing and definitive recommendations are still to be made on the use of these diets to improve glycaemic control.

Parenteral nutrition

- Similar PN regimens can be used as those given to non-diabetics.
- May require extra potassium and phosphate, according to blood glucose control.
- If insulin is added to the PN bag, approximately 30% will bind to the plastic. In general, insulin should be given by a separate infusion pump.

Hyperglycaemia

- Hyperglycaemia may occur secondary to illness or infection, overfeeding (especially with PN), medication (e.g. corticosteroids), insufficient insulin or OHAs, or volume depletion.
- Aim to keep blood glucose between 5.5–11.0 mmol/l in the catabolic patient and between 5.5–8.5 mmol/l once stable.
- Adjust diabetes medication rather than reducing the volume of feed – it is important to meet the patient's nutritional requirements.
- Where blood glucose levels are >11 mmol/l, review diabetes treatment before increasing feed rate.
- Short-term complications of hyperglycaemia include hypertriglyceridaemia, risk of dehydration and hyperosmolar non-ketotic coma/ketosis and impaired immune function with increased risk of infection, such as catheter sepsis.

Hypoglycaemia

- Hypoglycaemia may occur as a consequence of:
  - inappropriate use of diabetic medication
  - interruption to nutritional support
  - vomiting in patients on insulin or sulphonylureas
  - reduction in medication that causes hyperglycaemia, e.g. corticosteroids
  - underlying clinical condition, e.g. severe hepatitis.
- Aim to keep blood glucose >5.5 mmol/l.
- Treat immediately with:
  - 15–20 g oral carbohydrate where patient is able to swallow and has a functioning gut, e.g. Lucozade, non-diet fizzy drink, glucose tablets, Hypostop
  - a glucose drink *via* the NG tube/PEG where oral administration is not possible, or IV dextrose or IM/SC glucagon (1 mg) in exceptional circumstances
  - then maintain blood glucose within the target range by providing additional carbohydrate or reviewing diabetic medication.

Further reading

- Consensus roundtable on nutrition support in tube fed patients with diabetes (1998) Consensus statement. *Clin Nutr.* **17** (Suppl 2): 63–5.
- Coulston AM (1998) Clinical experience with modified enteral formulas for patients with diabetes. *Clin Nutr.* **17** (Suppl 2): 46–56.
- Wright J (2000) Total parenteral and enteral nutrition in diabetes. *Curr Opin Nutr Metabol Care.* **3**: 5–10.

Inflammatory bowel disease

There are two issues to consider – firstly, the nutritional support of patients who may be undernourished and/or have an acute illness; secondly, the matter of using nutrition as a primary therapy for inflammatory bowel disease (IBD). The latter is only really relevant in acute Crohn's disease (*see* below).

Acute ulcerative colitis

- Unless there is clinical concern regarding imminent surgery, e.g. toxic dilatation, patients should eat normally ± supplements if necessary. Dietary requirements are no different from those of anyone else with an acute illness. There is *no* need to rest the gut and hence PN is not necessary.
- Low fibre/low lactose diet may provide symptomatic relief – resume normal diet following acute phase.
- Patients requiring surgery should be managed in the usual way (*see* Chapter 6).

Acute Crohn's disease

- Many patients with a flare up of Crohn's are unwell and catabolic, and may have an underlying problem of malabsorption and weight loss. Nutritional status needs to be assessed in the normal way and diet ± oral supplements prescribed if appropriate (with dietetic advice).
- There is a considerable literature on the use of diets, both elemental and polymeric (*see* Chapter 5 for further details), as a *primary* treatment for acute Crohn's relapse. To summarise briefly the evidence in adults:
  - dietary therapy is no better than steroids
  - all studies have compared diet to steroids; none have combined the two, even though in practice many gastroenterologists do this
  - one benefit of dietary therapy is avoiding the side-effects of steroids and other immunosuppressive medication. However, for maximal efficacy, there has to be absolute compliance with the diet as the sole source of nutritional intake over many weeks (6–8), and many patients find this very difficult
  - colonic Crohn's is probably less responsive to dietary therapy than small intestinal disease
  - there is no difference in the efficacy of elemental and polymeric diets, but polymeric is more palatable and compliance generally better where taken orally (as opposed to *via* a feeding tube)

– there is probably a higher relapse rate after dietary treatment than after steroids
– it is still unclear what 'ingredient or ingredients' (if any) in the diets are effective.

The evidence for the use of dietary therapy in favour of steroids in adults therefore is currently not particularly strong and, although there are ardent advocates of this approach, they are in the minority. Many gastroenterologists, however, use diet as an adjunct to steroids in difficult cases or as sole therapy where steroids are contraindicated or refused.

- Where diet is not used as a therapeutic option, a normal diet ± supplements is all that is required for the majority of patients.
- PN is only necessary in some cases of fistulating or stricturing disease or in those with difficult post-operative complications. In the latter situation it is usual to involve colleagues with specialist surgical and nutritional experience, and further detail is beyond the scope of this book.

Chronic ulcerative colitis and Crohn's disease (i.e. remission)

- No particular nutritional requirements.
- Vitamin B_{12}, folate, calcium and vitamin D supplementation may be required.

Further reading

- Goh J and O'Morain C (2003) Nutrition and adult inflammatory bowel disease. *Aliment Pharmacol Ther.* **17**: 307–20.
- King TS, Woolner JT and Hunter JO (1997) Review article: the dietary management of Crohn's disease. *Aliment Pharmacol Ther.* **11**: 17–31.
- Song HK and Buzby GP (2001) Nutritional support for Crohn's disease. *Surg Clin North Am.* **81**: 103–15.

Liver disease

- Acute liver disease induces the same metabolic effects as any critical illness situation. The effect on nutritional status depends on the duration of the disease and the presence of any underlying chronic liver disease, which may have already compromised the patient's nutritional status.
- In patients with chronic liver disease, the most common type of malnutrition is that of a mixed protein–energy malnutrition.

Acute liver failure

Manage as for critical illness situation (*see* nutritional support in the critically ill patient, pp. 92–6).

Acute on chronic (decompensated) liver disease

- It was thought that protein restriction was necessary because of the risk of precipitating encephalopathy. However, these patients are catabolic, and protein restriction leads to greater muscle breakdown with the inherent risks of diminished skeletal and respiratory muscle function with consequent delay in mobilisation and increased incidence of chest infections. These issues outweigh the more theoretical argument surrounding encephalopathy, and therefore patients need high energy, high protein diets.
- However, because of the above described issues, liver 'friendly' diets have been formulated supplemented with branched chain amino acids in favour of the aromatic amino acids, which are thought to be more relevant in the genesis of encephalopathy. Numerous studies have been carried out to test their efficacy. The *only* indication for their use is where a standard protein-enriched diet worsens encephalopathy, providing other precipitating causes have been excluded, such as sepsis and bleeding.
- All that most patients will require is a high protein diet ± supplements (25–35 kcal/kg/day energy with 1.5 g/kg/day protein).
- Usually patients can eat normally.
- Tube feeding will be required if the patient is unable or unwilling to eat sufficiently. There is negligable risk to varices from a fine bore NG tube, and hence the presence of varices should not be a contraindication to NG feeding.
- Parenteral feeding should be reserved only for those not prepared to co-operate with oral or tube feeding.
- Fat-soluble vitamin supplementation plus zinc and selenium may be required.
- Decompensation secondary to alcohol, or where pre-existing malnutrition exists, requires a loading dose of Pabrinex or other vitamin B/C complex.
- The presence of ascites should lead to a salt (and fluid) restriction (60–80 mmol/l per day) unless there is significant renal impairment where more liberal fluid regimens may be more appropriate.

Chronic compensated (stable) liver disease

- These patients, especially those with an alcohol aetiology, may have mixed protein–energy malnutrition.
- There are no particular dietary requirements, although these patients may require standard oral supplementation if dietary intake is inadequate or there is pre-existing undernutrition.
- Fat-soluble vitamin supplementation plus zinc and selenium may be required.

Further reading

- Dudrick SJ and Kavic SM (2002) Hepatobiliary nutrition: history and future. *J Hepatobiliary Pancreat Surg.* **9**: 459–68.
- Florez DA and Aranda-Michel J (2002) Nutritional management of acute and chronic liver disease. *Semin Gastrointest Dis.* **13**: 169–78.
- Kondrup J and Muller MJ (1997) Energy and protein requirements of patients with chronic liver disease. *J Hepatol.* **27**: 239–47.

- Plauth M, Merli M, Kondrup J *et al.* (1997) ESPEN guidelines for nutrition in liver disease and transplantation. *Clin Nutr.* **16**: 43–55.

Short bowel syndrome

Chronic intestinal failure leading to the short bowel syndrome and its management is a complex clinical situation that should be managed by a multidisciplinary clinical team experienced with such patients. As such, a detailed description is beyond the scope of this book. The further reading list at the end of this section refers to appropriate texts.

What follows is a brief outline of the important and most relevant issues.

- Short bowel syndrome, the most common sequela of chronic intestinal failure, is where there is insufficient small intestine to allow adequate absorption of fluid, electrolytes and nutrients.
- The small intestine can be regarded as 'short' if its length is < 200 cm.
- The normal length of the small intestine ranges from 275–850 cm. Therefore in cases of surgical resection, it is essential that operating notes document the length of intestine *remaining* and not just the amount removed.
- Preservation of the ileocaecal valve is of great relevance, as it slows intestinal transit leading to increased absorption of water and electrolytes, and prevents bacterial colonisation of the small bowel (by inhibiting reflux of colonic content).
- Management depends on whether there is a jejuno-ileal resection and colectomy with an end jejunostomy, or whether there is a jejuno-colic anastamosis (*see* Figures 7.2a and 7.2b).

Causes of short bowel

- Ischaemia/infarction (most commonly due to superior mesenteric thrombosis).
- Crohn's disease/resection.
- Radiation.
- Volvulus.
- Tumours.

Management

Jejunostomy
- *See* Figure 7.2a and Tables 7.3 and 7.4.
- The biggest problem for these patients is with fluid and electrolyte balance rather than energy intake.
- *Fluid and electrolyte losses* are high with up to 4 l/day from intrinsic secretions alone (saliva, gastric and pancreatic).
  - Patients with > 100 cm jejunum usually have sufficient intestine to absorb more salt and water than they ingest and can be managed with oral sodium and water supplements without needing parenteral fluids – these are net 'absorbers'.

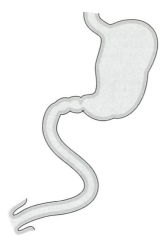

Figure 7.2a   End jejunostomy.

- – Patients with < 100 cm jejunum are unable to absorb sufficiently and lose more salt and water than they ingest orally. These patients therefore have a high-output jejunostomy and will require parenteral saline supplementation – these are net 'secretors'.
- Consumption of water and hypotonic fluid dilutes luminal contents and will exacerbate fluid losses. This occurs because jejunal sodium concentration needs to be maintained at approximately 90 mmol/l. If this is diluted by oral hypotonic fluid, sodium will diffuse into the lumen to correct the dilution. As a result, sodium (and water) is literally washed out of the body. Where jejunostomy losses are high, intake of water and hypotonic fluid should be kept to a minimum (< 500 ml/day), and instead isotonic/hypertonic fluids (sodium concentration > 90 mmol/l) should be encouraged, even though they are not very palatable.
- *Gastric acid secretion* usually increases due to lack of inhibitory hormones, which would normally be secreted from more distal small intestine. Not only will this increase the risk of peptic ulceration, but it will also inactivate gut hormones and lead to impaired absorption and greater diarrhoea. Gastric acid hypersecretion usually goes on for 3–6 months before returning to normal. High dose H_2 receptor antagonists or proton pump inhibitors are therefore indicated.
- *Anti-motility agents*, such as loperamide (4 mg qds), codeine phosphate (60 mg qds) and octreotide (50 μg twice daily SC or IV), can all help lessen gut losses.
- *Hypomagnesaemia* is a common problem. Low levels are due to loss of magnesium-absorbing sites (ileum, colon), secondary hyperaldosteronism due to salt and water losses (causes increased renal magnesium excretion), and free fatty acids in the gut lumen binding to orally ingested magnesium. Magnesium deficiency can lead to fatigue, depression, muscle weakness, tetany and convulsions. If supplementation is required there are either oral preparations (magnesium oxide 4 mmol capsules) or parenteral infusions. In addition, low magnesium can further exacerbate the problem by reducing the secretion and function of parathormone, which under normal circumstances promotes renal magnesium reabsorption and increases the formation of 1,25 hydroxycholecalciferol, which in turn increases intestinal absorption of magnesium (and

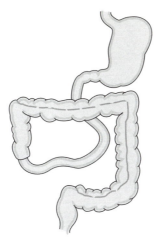

Figure 7.2b   Jejuno-colic anastamosis.

calcium). Therefore provision of 1-α cholecalciferol (1–9 μg daily) is a useful adjunct to magnesium supplementation.
- Providing at least one-third of energy intake can be absorbed, food intake can be 'normal'. Because of the malabsorption more energy needs to be consumed to maintain weight, and therefore often nutritional supplements are required. Because there is no colon there need be no restriction on fat intake. Elemental diets should *not* be used as they are hypertonic with low sodium content and will lead to net salt and water losses. If patients are unable to absorb sufficiently (usually < 100 cm jejunum) long-term PN will be required.
- Vitamin B$_{12}$ and D supplementation will be required.

Jejunum–colon patients
- *See* Figure 7.2b.
- If remaining jejunum is < 50 cm, these patients will require long-term parenteral feeding.
- If remaining jejunum is > 100 cm, they should be able to resume a normal diet without any need of supplements in the long term (although supplementation may be required in the short term while adaptation takes place).
- For those with 50–100 cm jejunum it is likely that oral diet + supplements will be adequate, but it may take several months for adaptation to occur to allow this.
- The colon retains its ability to absorb fluid and therefore these patients rarely get troubled with salt, water or magnesium losses.
- Dietary intake needs to be energy-rich because of the malabsorption. The diet should be carbohydrate and protein-rich and fat-poor. This will lessen malodorous steatorrhoea.
- Renal oxalate stones can occur. In the normal situation calcium binds oxalate in the gut and prevents its absorption. In the short bowel calcium will preferentially bind to free fatty acids leaving oxalate ions unbound and free for absorption in the colon. Diet therefore needs to be low in oxalate (i.e. avoiding rhubarb, spinach, beetroot, peanuts).
- Where diarrhoea occurs, loperamide and codeine phosphate can be helpful.

Table 7.3 Management of short bowel with jejunostomy

Problem	Presentation	Management	Monitoring
Correct dehydration	Presents with: ↓ body weight systolic hypotension ↓ urine output ↑ urea/creatinine	IV saline and nil by mouth for 24–48 hr initially. This ↓ thirst Restrict oral hypotonic fluids <500 ml/day Oral glucose/saline solution (Na >90 mmol/l. At least 1 litre/day should be encouraged. Palatability improved with chilling or flavoured with fruit juice Salt should be added to enteral feeds to make concentration up to 100 mmol/l	Daily weight + accurate fluid balance Urinary Na every 2 days initially. 0–5 mmol/l indicates depletion Aim at urine volume >800 ml/day + Na concentration of >20 mmol/l
↓ Stomal output	Exclude other causes of a high output stoma, e.g. sepsis, enteritis, partial/intermittent bowel obstruction, recurrent disease (e.g. Crohn's), abrupt cessation of drugs (e.g. steroids, loperamide)	Loperamide (up to 24 mg/day) Codeine phosphate (60 mg qds) ↓ Gastric acid with H$_2$ receptor antagonists (e.g. cimetidine 400 mg qds) or proton pump inhibitors (e.g. omeprazole 40 mg od) Octreotide (50 μg twice daily IV or SC	Daily (meticulous) fluid balance charts

Hypomagnesaemia	Fatigue, muscle weakness, ataxia, cardiac arrhythmias, convulsions	Oral Mg (12 mmol Mg oxide nocte) or IV Mg sulphate if necessary 1-α cholecalciferol (1–9 μg daily)	Serum Mg every 2 days initially. 1–2 per week thereafter
Energy intake	Undernutrition presents gradually	<100 cm jejunum for IV feeding >100 cm jejunum for high energy, high protein diet. No fat restriction necessary. If oral diet ± supplements insufficient, may need enteral tube feeding via NG or PEG, e.g. at night	Body weight and anthropometric measurements. If weight falls or cannot be regained despite maximal oral/enteral feeding IV feeding will be required
Vitamin, minerals and trace elements	*See* Table 4.6 for clinical features of deficiencies	Particular attention needs to be given to: Fat-soluble vitamins (A, D, E, K) Selenium B_{12} Essential fatty acids (treated by rubbing sunflower oil into skin)	Regular monitoring required

Table 7.4 Problems with a short bowel

	Jejunostomy	Jejunum–colon
Water and sodium depletion	Very common	Uncommon
Diet	High energy, no fat restriction necessary	High energy, fat restriction
Magnesium supplements	Usually required	Often not required
Renal oxalate stones	No	Yes
Gallstones (pigment)	Approx 50%	Approx 50%

Further reading

- Nightingale JMD (ed) (2001) *Intestinal Failure*. Greenwich Medical Media, London.
- Ukleja A, Scolapio JS and Buchman AL (2002) Nutritional management of short bowel syndrome. *Semin Gastrointest Dis*. **13**: 161–8.
- Vanderhoof JA and Langnas AN (1997) Short bowel syndrome in children and adults. *Gastroenterology*. **113**: 1767–78.

Acute stroke

- ~30% patients hospitalised with acute stroke are malnourished.
- Malnutrition is multifactorial and can occur because of impaired swallow, reduced level of consciousness, poor mobility, arm/facial weakness, depression, ill-fitting dentures.
- Those patients with a safe swallow should be fed with appropriate diets and given any necessary assistance to eat.
- Up to 50% of hospitalised stroke patients are unable to swallow safely on admission. Dysphagia is associated with greater severity of stroke and has a 6 week mortality of approximately 50%.
- For patients with unsafe swallow, tube feeding needs to be considered (*see* Figure 7.3).
- Swallow will recover in many patients over the first 2–4 weeks sufficiently to allow thickened fluids and food to be taken safely. Speech and language therapists will advise on the correct texture and consistencies for diet and fluids.
- While adequate feeding is a necessary part of patient care, neither nutritional supplementation for those able to swallow nor enteral tube feeding for those who cannnot has any effect on overall outcome.
- For those in whom tube feeding is considered, very careful thought has to be given to the appropriateness of such a step (*see* Chapter 12 for further discussion).

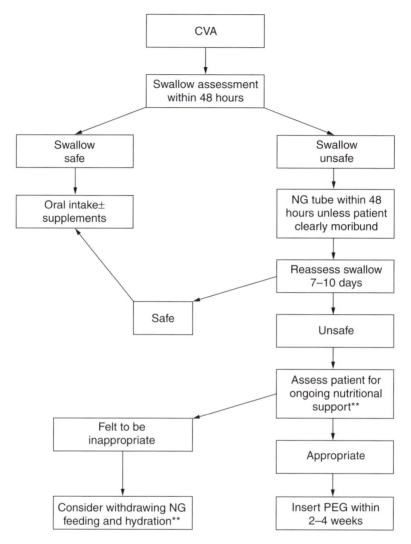

Figure 7.3 Pathway for nutritional management of acute stroke.

Further reading

- Blackmer J (2001) Tube feeding in stroke patients: a medical and ethical perspective. *Can J Neurol Sci.* **28**: 101–6.
- Dennis M (2000) Review: nutrition after stroke. *Br Med Bull.* **56**: 466–75.
- Gariballa SE and Sinclair AJ (1998) Assessment and treatment of nutritional status in stroke patients. *Postgrad Med J.* **74**: 395–9.
- Perry L and McLaren S (2003) Nutritional support in acute stroke: the impact of evidence-based guidelines. *Clin Nutr.* **22**: 283–93.

Hyperemesis gravidarum

- Severe nausea and vomiting persisting after 14th week of pregnancy. Occurs in 2% of pregnancies.
- Risk of dehydration, electrolyte imbalance and ketonuria.
- Where weight loss exceeds 5% of pre-pregnancy weight hospitalisation is usually required.
- IV fluid and electrolytes, anti-emetic drugs ± steroids with psychological support are usually effective, but if intractable vomiting and metabolic upset persist nutritional support will be required.
- Intragastric feeding is not to be recommended because of the risk of aspiration.

The choice is therefore between the following.

- *Post-pyloric feeding.*
  - NJ tube.
    - (i)   Self-propelling. Gastric motility is unaffected and so spontaneous trans-pyloric passage should be achievable in >80%.
    - (ii) Endoscopic placement.
  - PEGJ. Requires PEG. Although reported to be safe, because of more acceptable alternatives, there may be reluctance on the part of patient, obstetrician and endoscopist to utilise this route.
- *Parenteral feeding.* Attendant risks of line sepsis etc (*see* p. 68). Also likely to need prolonged hospitalisation to train and stabilise.

Further reading

- Hamaoui E and Hamaoui M (2003) Nutritional assessment and support during pregnancy. *Gastroenterol Clin North Am.* **32**: 59–121.
- Kuscu NK and Koyuncu F (2002) Hyperemesis gravidarum: current concepts and management. *Postgrad Med J.* **78**: 76–9.

PART 3

Children

CHAPTER 8

Paediatric nutritional assessment

Introduction

As in adult practice, nutritional assessment is used to:

- determine nutritional status and identify those likely to benefit from nutritional support
- determine goals of nutritional support
- act as a baseline against which nutritional management can be monitored.

Although there is no single way of defining undernutrition the factors detailed below are useful in identifying it.

If undernutrition is identified, or a child/infant is assessed to be at risk of becoming undernourished, it is essential that appropriate action is taken. Hospitals should have protocols in place to identify such patients and direct appropriate ongoing nutritional management, which will invariably involve dietitians ± nutrition teams.

Methods of assessment
Nutritional intake

A diet history should be taken from the parent or carer to assess current food/fluid intake, changes in appetite and risk factors (*see* nutritional screening, below). This together with feed/fluid charts kept by nursing staff should provide information on the nutritional intake of the child.

Some questions to ask when taking a feeding history:

- type of milk (infants: breast or formula; children: whole or semi-skimmed milk)
- if bottle fed – how much, how often and total feeds in 24 hours
- check feed preparation and technique if bottle fed
- meals and snacks – timing, quantity eaten
- textures – is the child eating age-appropriate foods?
- who feeds the child and where?
- does the child vomit – if yes, when, how often, how much?
- stools – consistency and frequency.

Weight/height/head circumference measurements

- Infants must be weighed naked and children in clean nappy/pants on calibrated scales with 10 g accuracy.
- Supine length must be measured in children under 2 years of age on a stadiometer with all head wear and socks/shoes removed. Standing height should be taken for children over 2 years of age.
- Head circumference is a useful measurement in children under 2 years of age, particularly if supine length is difficult to establish. Weight, height and/or head circumference measurements should be plotted on Cole 1995 centile charts to assess overall growth progress.
- Weight faltering can be taken generally as a two major centile difference to the height/head circumference plot.
- In addition, growth failure can be assessed using the Child Growth Foundation 1996 thrive lines whereby serial plots can be compared with the steepness of the thrive lines.
- Separate centile charts are available for children with Down's syndrome.

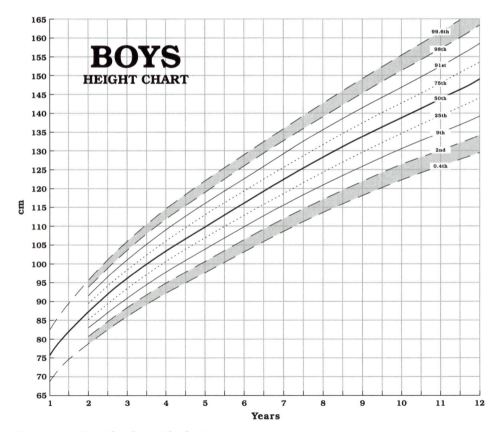

Figure 8.1 Boys' height centile chart.

Normal birth weight in the UK is 3.3–3.5 kg. There is usually some weight loss in the first 5–7 days usually up to 10%, which is regained by 10–14 days, i.e. there is no net weight gain during the first 10–14 days of age.

Expected weight gain for infants:

- <2 kg 15–28 g/kg/day
- >2 kg to 3 months of age 30 g/day
- 4–6 months of age 150 g/week
- 7–9 months of age 100 g/week
- 10–12 months of age 50–75 g/week.

A child following the 50th centile will gain approximately 2.5 kg in the second year and then 2 kg each year until puberty.

Percentage weight loss

This is a useful measurement of nutritional status in the absence of oedema and ascites. Rapid weight alterations are likely to be fluid and not body mass.

$$\text{Percentage weight loss} = \frac{(\text{usual weight kg} - \text{actual weight kg})}{\text{usual weight kg}} \times 100$$

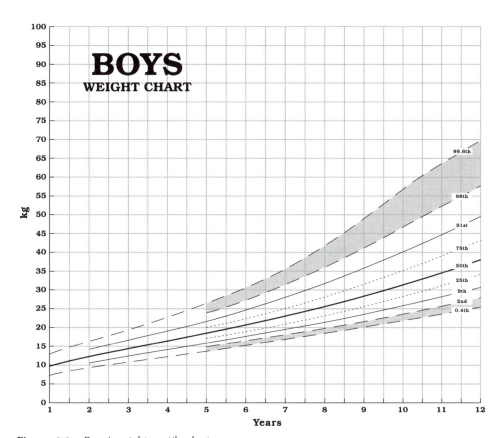

Figure 8.2 Boys' weight centile chart.

Interpretation of percentage weight loss (over 6–12 weeks):

- $<5\%$ – not significant (unless rapid or ongoing)
- 5–9% – not serious (unless rapid)
- 10–20% – clinically significant, requires nutritional support
- $>20\%$ – severe, requires aggressive nutritional support.

Body mass index

$$\text{BMI} = \frac{\text{weight kg}}{(\text{height m})^2}$$

This provides an indication of fatness or thinness. Age related centile charts are available which relate a child's fatness or thinness to his/her height and age (*see* Figures 8.1 to 8.4). Its use is limited in children for assessing nutritional status as it is an index, which enhances any measuring inaccuracies that may be present. Also there are simpler methods that can be used. BMI is therefore not an assessment of choice in paediatric practice.

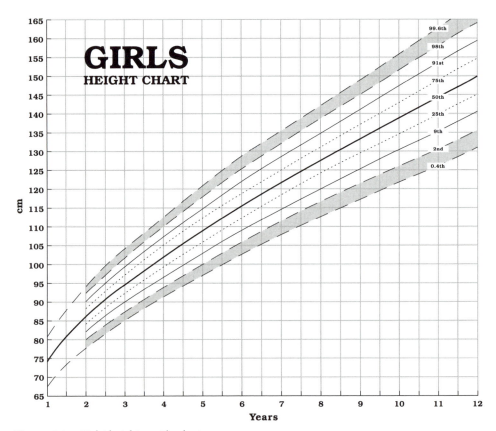

Figure 8.3   Girls' height centile chart.

Height for age and weight for height

- These figures are calculated using the Cole 1995 centile charts (*see* Figures 8.1 to 8.4) or the Cole's Growth rule (Child Growth Foundation).
- *Height for age* is calculated using the actual height of that child divided by the 50th centile for height of the age of the child concerned. For example:
  - girl aged 6.2 years is 93 cm actual height and 10 kg actual weight. The 50th centile height of a child aged 6.2 years is 117 cm.

$$\text{The \% height for age is } \frac{93}{117} \times 100 = 79.5\%$$

- *Weight for height* is calculated by dividing actual weight by weight age. To calculate this, the 50th centile age for the child's height is obtained (height age), and then the 50th centile weight for this height age (weight age). For example:
  - this same child of 6.2 years is 93 cm actual height and 10 kg actual weight. The 50th centile age of a child measuring 93 cm is 2.7 years. Referring to the charts of a 2.7 year old, the 50th centile weight is 14 kg (this is the weight

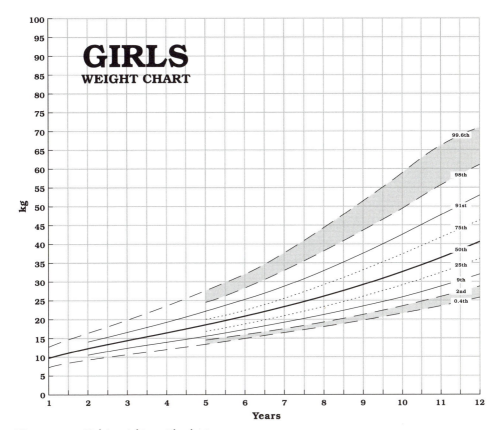

Figure 8.4 Girls' weight centile chart.

age). To calculate the % weight for height, the actual weight is divided by the weight age multiplied by 100, i.e.

$$\frac{10}{14} \times 100 = 71\%$$

Classification of undernutrition from weight for height and height for age measurements.

- 80–90% weight for height = grade 1 acute undernutrition (wasting).
- 70–80% weight for height = grade 2 acute undernutrition (wasting).
- <70% weight for height = grade 3 acute undernutrition (wasting).
- 90–95% height for age = grade 1 chronic undernutrition (stunting ± wasting).
- 85–90% height for age = grade 2 chronic undernutrition (stunting ± wasting).
- <80% height for age = grade 3 chronic undernutrition (stunting ± wasting).

Anthropometry

- Mid upper arm circumference (MUAC) is a useful measurement in <5 years of age, particularly if an accurate weight is difficult to establish due to oedema/ascites or solid tumour. It measures upper arm muscle and fat stores, and can establish an approximate weight centile through reference tables (*see* Table 8.1).

Table 8.1 Percentiles of MUAC for children (mm)

Age (yrs)	Centile						
	5	10	25	50	75	90	95
1–1.9	142	146	150	159	170	176	183
2–2.9	141	145	153	162	170	178	185
3–3.9	150	153	160	167	175	184	190
4–4.9	149	154	162	171	180	186	192
5–5.9	153	160	167	175	185	195	204
6–6.9	155	159	167	179	188	209	228
7–7.9	162	167	177	187	201	223	230
8–8.9	162	170	177	190	202	220	245
9–9.9	175	178	187	200	217	249	257
10–10.9	181	184	196	210	231	262	274
11–11.9	186	190	202	223	244	261	280
12–12.9	193	200	214	232	254	282	303
13–13.9	194	211	228	247	263	286	301
14–14.9	220	226	237	253	283	303	322
15–15.9	222	229	244	264	284	311	320
16–16.9	244	248	262	278	303	324	343
17–17.9	246	253	267	285	308	336	347
18–18.9	245	260	276	297	321	353	379

Table 8.2 Sample paediatric screening tool

NAME:	WARD:
HOSPITAL NO:	DATE:
DOB:	
WEIGHT:	CENTILE:
HEIGHT/LENGTH:	HEAD CIRC:
CENTILE:	CENTILE:

Please circle relevant score. Only select one score from each section. Select the highest score that applies.

		Score
1	*Anthropometry*	
	No weight loss	0
	Usual weight in health (kg):	
	Present weight (kg):	
	Weight loss > 10% in last 3 months?	2
	On centile charts is weight plot 1 major centile below height plot?	2
	On centile charts is weight plot 2 major centiles below height plot?	4
	On centile charts is weight plot 3 or 4 major centiles below height plot?	6
2	*Appetite*	
	Good appetite, manages most of 3 meals daily (or equivalent)	0
	Poor appetite, poor intake − leaving > half of meals provided (or equivalent)	2
	Appetite nil or virtually nil, unable to eat. NBM (no food for > 4 meals)	3
3	*Nutritional intake*	
	No difficulties in eating, able to eat independently	
	No diarrhoea or vomiting	0
	Problems handling food, e.g. needs special cutlery	
	Vomiting/frequent regurgitation possetting/mild diarrhoea	1
	Difficulty swallowing, requiring modified consistency	
	Problems with chewing affecting intake, slow to feed	
	Vomiting and/or diarrhoea 1–2 times daily	
	Needs help with feeding (e.g. physical handicap)	2
	Unable to take food orally	
	Unable to swallow (complete dysphagia)	
	Severe vomiting and/or diarrhoea (> 2 times daily)	
	Malabsorption	3
4	*Stress factor*	
	No stress factor: e.g. admission for investigations only	0
	Mild: Minor surgery, minor infection	1
	Moderate: Chronic disease	
	Major surgery/infections	
	Fractures	
	Pressure sores	
	Inflammatory bowel disease	
	Other GI disease	2
	Severe: Multiple injuries	
	Multiple fractures/burns	
	Multiple deep pressure sores, severe sepsis	
	Carcinoma/malignant disease	3
	TOTAL	

COMPLETE ON ADMISSION AND WEEKLY IF PATIENT'S CONDITION HAS CHANGED

Score		Action
0–3	*Low risk*	No action necessary
		Check weight at least weekly
4–5	*Needs monitoring*	Check weight at least weekly
		Encourage with eating and drinking
		Replace missed meals with supplements
		(Check with dietitian if on a special diet)
		Repeat score after one week and ask medical staff to
		refer patient to dietitian if no improvement
6–15	*High risk*	Ask medical staff to refer patient to dietitian

Also refer to dietitian if patient needs advice about a therapeutic diet

- Skinfold thickness requires training to be carried out accurately, but is a measure of fat stores in the area measured. Triceps, supra iliac and subscapular skinfolds are the most commonly used.
- Triceps skinfold can be used in conjunction with MUAC to calculate mid arm muscle circumference (MAMC) – *see* Chapter 3 for further details. UK reference centile charts are available for triceps and subscapular skinfold measurements.

Clinical assessment

The following could affect a child's nutritional needs.

- Medical condition of the child.
- Is the gut functioning normally?
- Are there increased losses, e.g. vomiting, diarrhoea, high stoma output?
- Are there increased requirements, e.g. malabsorption, pyrexia, stress?
- Nutritional deficiencies, e.g. iron deficiency anaemia.
- Physical appearance, e.g. thin, sparse hair, dry flaky skin, angular stomatitis.
- Abnormal nail shapes, such as spooning (koilonychias) indicative of iron deficiency.
- Persistent nappy rash resistant to treatment – may be an indication of zinc deficiency.

Biochemical measurements

A number of whole blood, serum or blood cell tests can be done to indicate nutritional status but these are not available routinely. *See* Chapter 3 for further details.

Nutritional screening

Nutritional screening is a way of identifying patients who are undernourished or at risk of becoming undernourished and involves completing a form to assess nutritional status that is usually carried out at the point of hospital admission. Screening should be repeated at weekly intervals unless a child is identified as being at high risk, in which case the child should be referred to the dietitian. A national nutritional screening tool is currently being validated for use in paediatrics, but an example of (an unvalidated) one is shown in Table 8.2.

Further reading

- Shaw V and Lawson M (eds) (2001) *Clinical Paediatric Dietetics* (2e). Blackwell Science, Oxford.
- Wright CM, Booth IW, Buckler JMH *et al.* (2002) Growth Reference Charts for use in the United Kingdom. *Arch Dis Child.* **86**: 11–14.

CHAPTER 9

Paediatric nutritional requirements

Requirements of healthy children

There are very little data available on nutritional requirements in children and much is extrapolated from work done in the adult population.

- Dietary reference values (DRV) can be used as a baseline for the individual child (*see* Table 9.1). It is important to remember that the reference values are intended to be used for healthy populations.
- Estimated average requirements (EAR) are based on FAO/WHO/UNU 1985 values, and used as a basis for assessing energy requirements.
- Reference nutrient intakes (RNI) are the values quoted for protein, vitamin and mineral requirements.
- Saturated fatty acids should be 11% of total dietary energy. Essential fatty acids: linoleic acid should be a minimum of 1% total dietary energy and α linolenic acid be a minimum of 0.2% total dietary energy.
- There are no specific recommendations for non-starch polysaccharides (NSP) or fibre in children but frequently the Williams *et al.* 1995 'age + 5' rule is used to obtain a daily value. For example a 4 year old should have NSP intake of $4 + 5 = 9$ g NSP daily.

Requirements of sick children

A general guide to nutritional requirements in sick children is given in Table 9.2. Examples of 'high' requirements would be burns ($< 10\%$), liver disease, inflammatory bowel disease, diarrhoea. Examples of 'very high' requirements would be critical illness, burns ($> 10\%$), multiple trauma. In very underweight children, it is more appropriate to use requirements based on weight age rather than actual age.

Requirements of children with low energy expenditure

Children with low energy expenditure, such as severely disabled children, are particularly at risk from overfeeding and excessive weight gain. A percentage

Table 9.1   Summary table of DRV

Age	Weight (kg)	Fluid (ml/kg)	Energy (kcal/d) (EAR)	Protein (g/d) (RNI)	Sodium (mmol/d) (RNI)	Potassium (mmol/d) (RNI)	Vit C (mg) (RNI)	Calcium (mmol/d) (RNI)	Iron (µmol/d) (RNI)
Males									
0–3 m	5.1	150	545	12.5	9	20	25	13.1	30
4–6 m	7.2	130	690	12.7	12	22	25	13.1	80
7–9 m	8.9	120	825	13.7	14	18	25	13.1	140
10–12 m	9.6	110	920	14.9	15	18	25	13.1	140
1–3 y	12.9	95	1230	14.5	22	20	30	8.8	120
4–6 y	19	85	1715	19.7	30	28	30	11.3	110
7–10 y	–	75	1970	28.3	50	50	30	13.8	160
11–14 y	–	55	2220	42.1	70	80	30	25	200
15–18 y	–	50	2755	55.2	70	90	40	25	200
Females									
0–3 m	4.8	150	515	12.5	9	20	25	13.1	30
4–6 m	6.8	130	645	12.7	12	22	25	13.1	80
7–9 m	8.1	120	765	13.7	14	18	25	13.1	140
10–12 m	9.1	110	865	14.9	15	18	25	13.1	140
1–3 y	12.3	95	1165	14.5	22	20	30	8.8	120
4–6 y	17.2	85	1545	19.7	30	28	30	11.3	110
7–10 y	–	75	1740	28.3	50	50	30	13.8	160
11–14 y	–	55	1845	42.1	70	70	35	20	260
15–18 y	–	50	2110	45.4	70	70	40	20	260

Table 9.2   General guide to requirements in sick children

	Preterm infants (< 37 weeks)	Infants (0–1 year)	Children
Energy	110–120 kcal/kg/d	High: 130–150 kcal/kg/d Very high: 150–220 kcal/kg/d	High: 120% EAR for age Very high: 150% EAR for age
Protein	< 1000 g < 27 weeks 3.6–3.8 g/kg/d > 1000 g > 27 weeks 3–3.6 g /kg/d	High: 3–4.5 g/kg/d Very high: 6 g/kg/d for up to 6 months to up to 10 g/kg/d for up to 1 year	High: 2 g/kg/d actual body weight
Sodium	0–7 days up to 1 mmol/kg/d 7 days–6 months 2–3 mmol/kg/d	High: 3 mmol/kg/d Very high: 4.5 mmol/kg/d	
Potassium		High: 3 mmol/kg/d Very high: 4.5 mmol/kg/d	

Table 9.3   Energy requirements for children with low energy expenditure

Age of child	Energy for maintenance and growth as % EAR (per kg actual body weight)
3 months	90%
9–12 months	85%
2–3 years	77%
4–5 years	71%
9–10 years	74%

of the EAR for age can be used to give a more realistic estimation of energy requirements, which is based on the WHO estimates of energy expenditure for maintenance, growth and activity (*see* Table 9.3).

Further reading

- Cocks A (ed) (2000) *Nutritional Requirements for Children in Health and Disease* (3e). Great Ormond Street Hospital for Children NHS Trust, London.
- Department of Health (1991) *Report on Health and Social Subjects No 41: Dietary Reference Values for Food Energy and Nutrients for the United Kingdom*. The Stationery Office, London.
- Thompson J (ed) (1997) *Nutritional Requirements of Infants and Young Children: practical guidelines*. Blackwell Science, Oxford.

CHAPTER 10

Methods of nutritional support

Introduction

The oral or enteral route is clearly the preferred method of feeding for children who have an adequately functioning gastrointestinal tract. Often it may simply involve increasing oral intake by use of food fortification, sip feeds or energy supplements. Where oral intake is not possible or inadequate but the gastrointestinal tract is functioning, tube feeding will be necessary.

The indications for the various routes of nutritional support are little different in principle to that of adult practice, and the illustration (*see* Figure 5.1) is worth referring to.

This book only deals with nutritional support in the acute hospital setting and will not be detailing any issues relating to nutritional support in the home or community.

Oral nutritional support

Indications for the use of oral/enteral nutritional support in children are listed in Table 10.1.

Food

Minimal interruption to meal times is of key importance. Nursing and medical staff must ensure this occurs wherever possible.

The type of nutritional support can be oral, if safe, by using extra snacks in addition to the hospital menu, or by fortifying foods with grated cheese, natural yoghurt/fromage frais, milk powder, double cream, olive oil, butter/polyunsaturated margarine, sugar/honey/syrup, or jam. The availability of 'snack boxes' from the 'Better Hospital Food' initiative ensures children that have missed a meal, due to their admission time or a procedure, get adequate food. In addition, the ward area should be conducive to eating/drinking, as suggested by the *Essence of Care* benchmarking document, so food should be presented nicely with child friendly crockery and cutlery in an area away from invasive procedures and distractions.

Table 10.1 Indications for use of oral/enteral nutritional support in children

Indication	Examples
Impaired suck, chew and swallow	Prematurity Cerebral palsy Neurodegenerative diseases Orofacial malformations Intensive care/ventilated patients
Breathlessness on feeding	Congenital heart disease Respiratory disease
Disordered appetite	Cachexia associated with chronic disease/malignancy Primary appetite disorder
Increased energy requirements	Cystic fibrosis Congenital heart disease Burns/trauma Liver disease Acquired immunodeficiency syndrome
Continuous supply of nutrients required	Short bowel syndrome Protracted diarrhoea Glycogen storage disorder
Unpalatability of specialised feeds	Crohn's disease Multiple food allergy/intolerance

Oral supplements

- The use of nutritional supplements (*see* Table 10.2) should be limited to those who are unable to meet their nutritional requirements through normal food and drink. This can be assessed by reviewing recent weight gain/growth, a nutritional screening tool (if available) or by a dietitian reviewing dietary assessment.
- Inappropriate use of nutritional supplements is associated with higher prescribing costs.
- There is a wide range of nutritional supplements available from powders to semi-solids to liquids (*see* Table 10.2). Some are nutritionally complete and can be taken as a sole source of nutrition and some are only designed to supplement the diet. Care has to be taken when using nutritionally complete supplements to ensure it complements current dietary intake and that there is not an excessive intake of any macro- or micronutrients.
- The patient's clinical condition may influence the choice of product, e.g. renal insufficiency will require caution with protein and electrolyte content.

Further reading

- Allison SP (ed) (1999) *Hospital Food as a Treatment. A report by a working party of the British Association for Parenteral and Enteral Nutrition.* BAPEN, Maidenhead.

Table 10.2 Types of paediatric nutritional supplements. (Examples have been given of some of the common supplements at the time of going to print. Some manufacturers state that their paediatric feeds are nutritionally complete for children over 6 years up to 30 kg in weight. Check individual company data, *BNF* and *MIMS* for up-to-date advice)

Product	Description	Approximate composition per item					
		Energy (kcal)	Protein (g)	Cho (g)	Fat (g)	Na (mmol)	K (mmol)
Glucose polymer powder (e.g. Polycal, Maxijul, Caloreen, Polycose) No age limit	*Calorie supplement only* Mixed into virtually any drink or moist food NB: Not suitable for diabetics Prescribable	Per 100 g Tasteless powder	380	–	95.0	–	Tr	Tr
Glucose polymer liquid (e.g. Polycal Liquid, Maxijul Liquid) No age limit	*Calorie supplement only* 200 ml bottle/Tetrabrik Sweet, cordial sip feed Diluted with equal parts of water NB: Not suitable for diabetics Prescribable	Apple Blackcurrant Lemon Orange Neutral	494	–	124.0	–	<0.3	<0.03
Duocal Super Soluble (Scientific Hospital Supplies) No age limit	*Calorie supplement only* 450 g can – powder Mixed into virtually any drink or moist food. Mixture of fat and carbohydrate Prescribable	Per 100 g: 490	490	–	72.7	27.3	<0.2	<0.1
1 kcal/ml sip feed (e.g. Paediasure [Abbott]) Age limit Use for children 8–30 kg	*Nutritionally complete* 200 ml carton with straw, ready-to-drink, milk-based sip feed. Serve chilled or at room temperature Prescribable	Chocolate Vanilla Strawberry Banana	200	5.6	22.2	10.0	5.22	5.64

Table 10.2 (continued)

Product	Description	Approximate composition per item					
		Energy (kcal)	Protein (g)	Cho (g)	Fat (g)	Na (mmol)	K (mmol)
1 kcal/ml sip feed with fibre (e.g. Paediasure Fibre [Abbott]) Age limit Use for children 8–30 kg	Nutritionally complete Details as above except contains approx 1.1 g fibre — Vanilla Strawberry Banana	200	5.6	22.2	10.0	5.22	5.64
1.5 kcal/ml sip feed (e.g. Fortini* [Nutricia], Frebini Energy Drink** [Fresenius], Paediasure Plus** [Abbott], Resource Junior*[1] [Novartis]) Age limit * Use from 1–6 years of age (8–20 kg) ** Children 8–30 kg	Nutritionally complete 200 ml Tetrabrik carton with straw 1.5 kcal/ml energy dense, ready to drink milk-based sip feed Prescribable except[1] — Vanilla Strawberry Chocolate Banana	300	6.8	37.6	13.6	7.8	8.4
1.5 kcal/ml sip feed with fibre (e.g. Fortini Multifibre [Nutricia], Frebini Energy Fibre Drink [Fresenius]) Age limit Use from 1–6 years of age (8–20 kg)	Nutritionally complete Details as above except each carton contains 1.5 g fibre Prescribable — Vanilla Strawberry Chocolate Banana	300	6.8	37.6	13.6	7.8	8.4

NB: Adult sip feeds can be used for children with caution. Many products can be used from 3 years of age without dilution but company data should be checked before using these products to ensure suitability and correct usage.

- Department of Health (2000) *Better Hospital Food. The NHS Plan.* The Stationery Office, London.
- Department of Health (2001) *Essence of Care: Patient focused benchmarking for healthcare professionals.* The Stationery Office, London.
- Todd EA, Hunt P, Crowe PJ *et al.* (1984) What do patients eat in hospital? *Hum Nutr Appl Nutr.* **38**: 294–7.

Enteral feeding
Choice of enteral diets
Infants
- There is a number of different diets for infants with normal gut function (*see* Table 10.3).
- There are also several specialised infant formulas, based on modified protein, fat and/or carbohydrate and used for a variety of medical conditions from food allergy/intolerance to malabsorption (*see* Table 10.4).
- Specialised formulas do not come as ready-to-feed formulas. They must be prepared, following manufacturers' directions, in a clean environment, usually in a milk kitchen.

Children 1–6 years (8–20 kg)
- *See* Tables 10.5 and 10.6.
- Several ready-to-feed preparations are available.
- All those listed are clinically lactose free.

Children >6 years (21–45 kg)
- An enteral feed range is now available for 7–12 year olds (21–45 kg) from Nutricia (Tentrini). The Paediasure (Abbott) and Frebini (Fresenius) ranges are also available for children weighing 8–30 kg (age 1–10 approximately).
- Adult feeds can be used with caution in children over 6 years and over 20 kg in weight. Protein and some micronutrient intakes may be inappropriately high. Feeds with a protein concentration >6 g protein/100 ml are unsuitable for most children.

Routes for enteral feeding
See Table 10.7 for routes for enteral tube feeding in children.

Short-term feeding (<6 weeks)
- Fine bore nasoenteral tubes:
  - NG
  - NJ (e.g. if vomiting a problem).
- Double lumen nasoenteral tubes:
  - gastric aspiration + jejunal feeding (e.g. in gastroparesis).

Table 10.3   Enteral tube feeds for infants with normal gut function

Feed	Examples	Energy (kcal/100 ml)	Protein (g/100 ml)	Prescribable?	Indications
Breast milk		66 (mature)	1.3	N/A	First choice. Expressed breast milk is used. Nutritionally complete for term infants <6 months if given at suitable volume
Standard infant formula (ready-to-feed)	SMA Gold, Cow & Gate Premium, Farley's First Milk, Aptamil First	66	1.4	No	Whey-based infant formulas (as listed) are closest to breast milk Casein-based feeds, e.g. SMA White, C&G Plus, are available but rarely indicated in clinical practice Nutritionally complete for term infants <6 months if given at suitable volume
High energy infant formula (ready-to-feed)	SMA High Energy	91	2	Yes	Fluid restricted infants Higher nutritional requirements
	Infatrini	100	2.6	Yes	Suitable for term infants up to 8 kg body weight

These feeds all contain lactose.

Table 10.4 Specialised infant enteral feeds. (The following table is designed as a guide to the various formulas available and their indications. It is not an exhaustive list. More detailed information can be obtained from *Special Foods for Children*, 2002. They are nutritionally complete for infants <6 months if given at a suitable volume. For infants over 6 months the formula would need to be concentrated to provide all major nutrients.)

Feed	Protein source	Fat source	Indications (not exhaustive)
Soya formula: Prosobee, Infasoy, Farley's soya formula, Wysoy	Soya protein	LCT	Cow's milk protein intolerance <6 months, lactose intolerance
Nutramigen (Mead Johnson)	Hydrolysed protein	LCT	Malabsorption of whole protein with or without dissacharide intolerance Cow's milk protein intolerance <6 months
Pregestimil (Mead Johnson)	Hydrolysed protein	55% MCT	Malabsorption of whole protein with or without disaccharide intolerance Fat malabsorption, e.g. liver disease
Prejomin (Milupa)	Hydrolysed protein	LCT	Malabsorption of whole protein with or without disaccharide intolerance Cow's milk protein intolerance <6 months
Pepti-Junior (Cow & Gate)	Hydrolysed protein	50% MCT	Malabsorption of whole protein with or without disaccharide intolerance Fat malabsorption, e.g. biliary atresia Cow's milk protein intolerance <6 months
Pepdite (SHS)	Hydrolysed protein	LCT	Malabsorption of whole protein with or without disaccharide intolerance Cow's milk protein intolerance <6 months
MCT Pepdite (SHS)	Hydrolysed protein	75% MCT	Malabsorption of whole protein with or without disaccharide intolerance Fat malabsorption
Enfamil Lactofree (Mead Johnson)	Whole protein	LCT	Lactose intolerance, galactosaemia
SMA LF (SMA)	Whole protein	LCT	Lactose intolerance, galactosaemia
Caprilon* (SHS)	Whole protein	75% MCT	Fat malabsorption without protein or dissacharide intolerance, e.g. Alagille's syndrome
Monogen *(SHS)	Whole protein	90% MCT	Fat malabsorption without protein or dissacharide intolerance, chylothorax, lipoproteinaemia type I
Neocate (SHS)	Free amino acids	LCT (mostly)	Severe malabsorption or multiple food intolerance

* Not lactose free. LCT = long chain triglyceride. MCT = medium chain triglyceride.

Table 10.5 Whole protein enteral feeds for children aged 1–6 years (8–20 kg)*

Energy (kcal/100 ml)	Protein (g/100 ml)	Na (mmol/100 ml)	K (mmol/100 ml)	With fibre?	Examples
75	1.7	2.6	2.8	Yes	Nutrini Low Energy Multi Fibre (Nutricia)
100	2.5–2.8	2.6	2.8	No	Paediasure* (Abbott) Nutrini (Nutricia) Frebini Original (Fresenius) Sondalis Junior (Nestle)
100	2.5–2.8	2.6	2.8	Yes	Paediasure Fibre* (Abbott) Nutrini Multi Fibre (Nutricia) Frebini Original Fibre* (Fresenius) Novasource Junior (Novartis)
150	4.1–4.2	3.9	4.6	No	Paediasure Plus* (Abbott) Frebini Energy (Fresenius) Nutrini Energy (Nutricia) Isosource Junior (Novartis)
150	4.1–4.2	3.9	4.6	Yes	Paediasure Plus Fibre* (Abbott) Nutrini Energy Multi Fibre (Nutricia)

*Some manufacturers now state that their paediatric feeds are nutritionally complete for children over 6 years up to 30 kg in weight. Check individual company data for recommendations for use.

Table 10.6 Specialised enteral feeds for children >1 year of age or >8 kg

Age	Type of feed	Composition per 100 ml						
		Energy (kcal)	Protein (g)	CHO (g)	Fat (g)	Na (mmol)	K (mmol)
1+ yr	*Peptide based*						
	Pepdite 1+ (Scientific Hospital Supplies)	85	2.76	3.46	11.4	1.82	2.64
	MCT Pepdite 1+ (Scientific Hospital Supplies)	91	2.8	3.60	11.8	1.8	2.6
6+ yr	Peptisorb (Nutricia Clinical Care)	100	4.0	17.6	1.7	3.5	3.6
	Peptamen (Nestlé)	100	4.0	12.7	3.7	3.2	3.5
	Perative (Abbott)	130	6.7	17.7	3.7	4.5	4.4
	Novasource Forte (Novartis)	150	6.0	18.3	5.9	3.7	3.5
	Survimed OPD (Fresenius)	100	4.5	15.0	2.6	6.0	4.0
1–5 yr	*Amino acid based*						
	Neocate Advance (Scientific Hospital Supplies)	100	2.5	3.5	14.6	2.6	3.0
5+ yr	Elemental 028 Extra (Scientific Hospital Supplies)	85.4	2.5	3.49	11.0	2.66	2.38

Table 10.7 Routes for enteral tube feeding in children

Type	Indications	Size	Complications	Specific care
NG Polyvinyl chloride tubes	Short term – bolus or continuous feeding Functioning GI tract but child unable to meet requirements with diet or supplements (see Table 10.1)	5 FG – neonates 6 FG – babies and small children 8 FG – older children (use of thickened feeds)	See p. 42 Tubes stiffen over time Sinusitis can be a problem	Insertion and site verification – see Table 10.8 Requires regular flushing with water to prevent blockage or bacterial contamination
Polyurethane fine bore NG tubes Made of soft polyurethane or silicone elastomer Fine bore tubes have stylets to give tube rigidity when passing	Long-term feeding Older children can be taught how to insert tube	5 FG – neonates 6 FG × 22 inch – babies 8 FG × 22 inch and 8 FG × 36 inch – useful size when using thickened feeds	High risk of tracheal intubation when inserting tube, if child is ventilated or has impaired swallow Displaceable if child prone to vomiting. (Weighted tubes no better) Tube prone to collapsing down when aspirating Can block if not flushed regularly	Insertion and site verification – see Table 10.8 Requires regular flushing using 50 ml syringe to prevent blockages Prior to insertion must ensure guide wire can be freely removed
Gastrostomy tubes Medical grade silicone material, ideally bio-compatible and flexible for patient comfort Should have retention discs on abdominal wall Gastric balloon should expand evenly	Used following surgical procedure (Stamm operation for insertion of a gastrostomy)	10 FG – younger children 12–14 FG – older children 16 FG	Can migrate into duodenum if inflation port of balloon is over-filled or if retention disc is not secured Low volume balloons are used in paediatrics (up to 5 ml) Skin problems, infection, leakage and granulation tissue Tube must be replaced within a few hours if accidentally removed, as stoma closes very quickly	See p. 53 Site cleaned daily and dried thoroughly Dressings not required unless site infected Vent tube and allow air to escape prior to child being fed Check placement using pH paper prior to use (pH 3–4)

PEG Made of pliable bio-compatible silicone Bumper bar helps to resist inadvertent removal and migration	Short- or long-term feeding As per NG tubes, plus congenital abnormalities such as oesophageal atresia or tracheo–oesophageal fistula	9 FG – younger children 15 FG – older children	*See* p. 53 Previous abdominal surgery can prevent use due to adhesions Removal of PEG is dependent on individual design Usually removed endoscopically in children under anaesthetic	*See* p. 53 Clean site daily Rotate tube daily Vent tube prior to use Check placement using pH paper prior to use (pH 3–4)
Skin level low profile devices (buttons)	Long-term feeding Replaced as per manufacturer's instructions – usually 4–6 monthly	12, 14, 16 FG Shaft length sizes: 1.5, 1.7, 2.0, 2.3, 2.5, 2.7, 3.0, 3.5, 4.0	Similar to PEG Leakage of gastric contents due to failure of anti-reflux valve	Rotate skin level device daily Clean site daily Extension sets required to access button for feeding
Post-pyloric feeding (NJ/jejunostomy)	Persistent vomiting or severe delayed gastric emptying, pulmonary aspiration Jejunostomy for long-term feeding		*See* pp. 50, 58, 59 NJ complications as per NG Jejunostomy: pain, stomal infection	Continuous feeding required pH paper required to check placement

Longer-term feeding (>6 weeks)

- Gastrostomies:
  - PEG (most common)
  - surgical gastrostomy (e.g. PEG technically not feasible)
  - fluoroscopic percutaneous gastrostomy
  - laparoscopic gastrostomy.
- Duodenostomy:
  - percutaneous endoscopic duodenostomy.
- Jejunostomy:
  - surgical jejunostomy
  - PEJ
  - jejunal tube inserted *via* PEG
  - needle catheter jejunostomy
  - cuffed tube jejunostomy
  - SC jejunostomy.

Practical considerations for enteral feeding

How to pass and care for an NG tube

- *See* Table 5.4 (adult section) for the general principles of NG tube insertion. However, where local policy/guidelines exist these should be referred to.
- Verification of correct siting of tube – *see* Table 10.8.
- Check for safe positioning of NG tube:
  - following initial insertion
  - prior to a bolus feed
  - following a vomit or a paroxysm of coughing
  - when symptoms suggest feed aspiration (coughing, choking, tachypnoea, wheezing)
  - when receiving a child moved from another clinical area
  - 12 hourly for children on continuous feeds
  - 4 hourly in infants and newborns on continuous feeds.
- Management of blocked tube – *see* Table 5.6.

Method of feeding

- *See* Table 10.9 for commonly used regimens and their indications.
- The type of regimen will depend on:
  - type of tube
  - oral feeding (maintenance and development of oral feeding skills should always be considered if oral feeding is safe for the child)
  - gastrointestinal function: reflux/vomiting, following gut resection, diarrhoea.
- If the tube feeding is to be continued at home, the practical aspects for the family must be carefully considered.

Patient monitoring

Children receiving enteral nutritional support require frequent monitoring to ensure their changing nutritional, developmental and psychological needs are met.

Table 10.8   How to confirm correct NG tube position. (Refer to local policy/ protocols if available)

Confirmatory test result	Action
Positive aspiration of gastric contents (blue litmus turns pink or pH < 4) and Correct external length of tube	Accept placement as correct
Unable to obtain/negative aspiration of gastric contents and Correct external length of tube	1 If possible offer drink to child and re-aspirate 2 Inject 2–5 ml air and re-aspirate 3 Inject 2–5 ml 0.9% sodium chloride, position child on their side and re-aspirate
Unable to obtain/negative aspiration of gastric contents and Incorrect external length of tube	Reposition tube to correct length and re-aspirate If no aspirate follow steps 1–3 above
Still unable to obtain/negative aspiration of gastric contents and Correct external length of tube	Confirm satisfactory placement by chest/abdominal X-ray or Remove tube and resite, then repeat confirmatory tests

NB: Following placement, the type, size and length of NG tube, and length of the external part of the tube should be clearly documented in the medical records.

A multidisciplinary approach to monitoring is important. Both hospital and community health professionals have a role in enteral feeding.

The following parameters may need to be assessed as often as daily initially, depending on the clinical condition of the child. Frequency of monitoring will reduce as stability on enteral feeds is achieved.

- Anthropometry (weight: minimum weekly; length/height: monthly).
- Feed tolerance and symptom control.
- Fluid input/output.
- Oral feeding.
- Biochemistry.

Other important points:

- *Nutritional requirements*:
  - should be reviewed as child gets older and gains weight
  - children receiving long-term nutritional support, particularly if as a sole source of nutrition, require nutritional and biochemical monitoring.
- *Oral feeding.* Liaise with nursing staff and speech therapist over oral stimulation if nothing is being taken orally. If there are concerns over safety of swallow,

Table 10.9 Regimens commonly used and their indications

Regimen	Comments
Bolus	3–4 hourly boluses commonly used in infant feeding Well tolerated if normal gut function Minimises equipment used at home (e.g. no feed pump) Stimulates bile flow Simulates 'feed' times Not indicated if feeding into the jejunum
Oral feeds with NG top-ups	Feed offered orally and remainder given as bolus *via* tube Useful when infants tire easily on feeds, e.g. congenital heart disease, poor oromotor skills
Continuously over 20 hours *via* feed pump if NG or over 24 hours if NJ/jejunostomy	Better tolerated in infants and children with gastric dysmotility or reflux Often used in short bowel as provides a continuous supply of nutrients to the adapting gut Continuous feeding is essential if feeding into the jejunum
Continuous feeding overnight	Useful if supplementing oral intake. Child can feed orally during the day Minimises disruption to daytime routine

never advise increasing oral intake without discussing with speech therapist and/or medical team first.

- *Development stage of child.* Involve other health professionals to ensure the psychological and practical needs of the child and family are met, e.g. health visitor, community nurses, school nurses.
- *Weaning from tube to oral feeding.* Never just stop enteral feeds in the hope of increasing oral intake. An incremental reduction of feeds in liaison with the multidisciplinary team (including carers) is recommended.

Drug administration *via* an enteral feeding tube

See p. 61.

Complications of enteral feeding

The major complications of enteral feeding itself, rather than related to the tube/route of delivery (*see* Table 10.7), are diarrhoea, nausea/vomiting and regurgitation/aspiration (*see* Table 10.10).

Table 10.10 Complications and management of enteral feeding complications

Symptom	Possible cause	Possible solution
Diarrhoea	Malabsorption/impaired gut function	Change to hydrolysed protein or elemental feed
	High feed osmolarity	Increase concentration of feed gradually
	Intolerance of bolus feeds	Smaller, more frequent bolus feeds or try feeding continuously using a feed pump
	Too fast an infusion rate	Slow infusion rate and increase as tolerated
	Feed contamination	Use closed systems wherever possible Always prepare other feed in a sterile environment
	Drugs, e.g. antibiotics, laxatives	Review drug prescription
Nausea/vomiting	Too fast an infusion rate	Trial continuous feeds
	Slow gastric emptying	Consider prokinetic drugs, jejunal feeding
	Psychological factors	Address behavioural feeding issues, refer to psychologist if appropriate
	Constipation	Maintain regular bowel motions with adequate fluid intake and laxatives. Trial of fibre feed
	Medicines given at the same time as feeds	Allow time between giving medicines and giving feeds or stop continuous feeds for a short time when medicines are given
Regurgitation and aspiration	Gastro-oesophageal reflux	Correct position, anti-reflux drugs, feed thickener, continuous infusion, post-pyloric feeding
	Dislodged tubes	Secure tube adequately and test position regularly
	Fast infusion rate	Slow infusion rate
	Intolerance of bolus feeds	Smaller, more frequent feeds or continuous infusion

Further reading

- ASPEN Board of Directors and Clinical Guidelines Task Force (2002) Guidelines for the Use of Parenteral and Enteral Nutrition in Adults and Paediatric Patients. *JPEN*. **26** (Suppl 1): 1SA–138SA.
- Davis A and Baker S (1996) The use of modular nutrients in pediatrics. *JPEN*. **20**: 228–36.
- Godbole P, Margabanthu G, Crabbe DC et al. (2002) Limitations and uses of gastrojejunal feeding tubes. *Arch Dis Child*. **86**: 134–7.
- Grant MJ and Martin S (2000) Delivery of enteral nutrition. *AACN Clin Issues*. **11**: 507–16.
- Holden C and MacDonald A (eds) (2000) *Nutrition and Child Health*. Harcourt Publishers, London.
- Holden C, MacDonald A, Ward M et al. (1997) Psychological preparation and support of children undergoing enteral nutrition: an evaluation. *Br J Nurs*. **6**: 376–85.

- MacDonald A, Holden C and Johnson T (2001) Paediatric enteral nutrition. In: J Payne-James, G Grimble and D Silk (eds) *Artificial Nutritional Support in Practice*. Greenwich Medical Media, London.
- Martin L and Cox S (2000) Enteral feeding: practice guidance. *Paediatr Nurs*. **12**: 28–33.
- Preedy V, Grimble G and Watson R (eds) (2001) *Nutrition in the Infant: problems and practical procedures*. Greenwich Medical Media, London.
- Sentongo T and Mascarenhas MR (2002) Newer components of enteral formulas. *Pediatr Clin North Am*. **49**: 113–25.
- *Special Foods for Children* (2002) Available from the Paediatric Group of the British Dietetic Association.

Parenteral feeding

Indications

- The most common indication for PN is reversal or prevention of malnutrition in 'gut failure' – impairment of gastrointestinal function sufficient to preclude adequate absorption of nutrients (*see* Table 10.11). General principles dictate that complete bowel rest should be avoided if possible. This is because enteral feeding even in small amounts helps maintain intestinal and pancreatic mass, stimulates bile secretion and splanchnic blood flow, protects against cholestasis and maintains gut barrier function.
- In many situations indications for PN are not absolute and clinical judgement is required. The involvement of a multidisciplinary nutritional care team in decision making and day-to-day management is therefore invaluable.
- Premature newborns represent the largest group of paediatric patients receiving PN, usually because immature gastrointestinal motor function prevents full enteral feeding over the first few weeks of life. In addition, rapid advancement

Table 10.11 Common indications for PN in children

Newborn	Unequivocal	Intestinal failure
		Functional immaturity
		NEC
		Short bowel syndrome
		Congenital abnormalities, e.g. gastroschisis, ileal atresia
	Equivocal	Respiratory failure requiring intermittent positive pressure ventilation
		Promotion of growth in preterm infants
		Prevention of NEC
Infants/children		Intestinal failure
		Post-operative gastrointestinal surgery
		Short bowel
		Protracted diarrhoea
		Chronic pseudo-obstruction

of enteral feeds has been associated with increased risk of necrotising entero-colitis (NEC) in this group of patients, a potentially devastating condition with high mortality and morbidity.

Routes, monitoring and complications

The information provided in the adult section (*see* p. 68) is applicable to paediatric practice.

Discontinuing PN

The decision to discontinue PN should be made only when there is documented evidence, preferably by a dietitian, that complete nutritional intake and absorption by the enteral route are possible, and when it is clear that no further imminent surgery, investigations or other stressful procedures are contemplated.

Children
Appetite often is reduced during PN, which may begin as a continuous infusion, but should then be administered during the night if possible to allow the child to participate in meal times during the day. Such 'cyclical' PN − 12 hours on 12 hours off − is also probably helpful in preventing cholestasis. If the child is not capable of eating/drinking, enteral tube feeding should commence. Oral or enteral tube intake should be accurately measured and the energy and protein intake of the PN scaled down accordingly as advised by the dietitian. During this period the PN should continue at full strength, the volume being gradually reduced as appropriate.

Once the child is managing approximately 75% of nutritional requirements by enteral/oral feeding, the PN should be discontinued. There will thus be an overlap between PN and enteral/oral feeding.

Infants
Enteral nutrition should commence by hourly bolus or continuous infusion (if not already established on enteral feeds) when weaning from PN. The PN should be scaled down according to volume of enteral nutrition tolerated, i.e. ml for ml. PN can cease once 75% of enteral requirements are tolerated. The PN volume should be scaled down proportionately between the amino acid/glucose infusion and the lipid to prevent ketosis and nutritional imbalance. Never reduce one infusion on its own. Discuss this with your paediatric pharmacist and dietitian.

In an ideal situation, the PN feeding line should stay *in situ* for at least 24 hours post-cessation of PN to ensure establishment on adequate enteral/oral feeding.

Further reading

- ASPEN Board of Directors and Clinical Guidelines Task Force (2002) Guidelines for the Use of Parenteral and Enteral Nutrition in Adults and Paediatric Patients. *JPEN.* **26** (Suppl 1): 1SA−138SA.
- Cooke RJ and Embleton ND (2000) Feeding issues in preterm infants. *Arch Dis Child Fetal Neonatal Ed.* **83**(3): F215−18.

- Duggan C, Rizzo C, Cooper A *et al.* (2002) Effectiveness of a clinical practice guideline for parenteral nutrition: a 5-year follow-up study in a pediatric teaching hospital. *JPEN.* **26**: 377–81.
- Harris J and Maguire D (1999) Developing a protocol to prevent and treat paediatric central venous catheter occlusions. *Intraven Nurs.* **22**: 194–8.
- Hodge D and Puntis JWL (2002) Diagnosis, prevention and management of catheter related blood stream infection during long term parenteral nutrition. *Arch Dis Child Fetal Neonatal Ed.* **87**: F21–4.
- Klavon S, Fuchs V, Gura K *et al.* (2002) New approaches to parenteral nutrition in infants and children. *J Paediatr Child Health.* **38**: 433–7.
- Meadows N (1998) Monitoring and complications of parenteral nutrition. *Nutrition.* **14**: 806–8.
- Pearson ML (ed) (1996) Guideline for Prevention of Intravascular Device Related Infections. *Am J Infection Control.* **24**: 262–93.
- Puntis JWL (2001) Paediatric parenteral nutrition. In: J Payne-James, GK Grimble and D Silk (eds) *Artificial Nutrition Support in Clinical Practice* (2e). Greenwich Medical Media, London.
- Shulman RJ and Phillips S (2003) Parenteral nutrition in infants and children. *J Paediatr Gastroenterol Nutr.* **36**: 687–707.
- Stringer M (1995) Vascular access. In: L Spitz and AG Coran (eds) *Pediatric Surgery* (5e). Chapman and Hall Medical, London.

CHAPTER 11

Nutritional support in disease-specific situations

Cystic fibrosis

- Cystic fibrosis affects 1 in 2500 live births in Caucasian populations.
- The main characteristics are pancreatic exocrine insufficiency and maldigestion, pulmonary disease, intestinal obstruction, liver disease, diabetes and infertility.
- Promoting better growth and nutrition is thought to improve survival.
- Dietary energy intake should be raised by around 20–30% through increasing dietary fat and sugar intake.
- Dietary supplements are frequently needed and overnight tube feeding common.
- 90% of patients have pancreatic exocrine insufficiency and require pancreatic enzyme replacement therapy.
- Diabetes is common with 2% of patients affected by 15 years of age, 12% by 25 years of age and 17% over 25 years of age.

Nutritional management

- Energy needs are increased in cystic fibrosis but individual requirements vary depending on age, activity and clinical status.
- Energy rich foods including full-cream milk, butter, cheese, meat, cakes and biscuits are encouraged.
- Recommended protein intake should represent 15% of the total energy intake to compensate for protein loss in stools and sputum; this can be achieved without specific supplementation.
- 35–40% of energy should be provided by fat.
- 45–50% of total energy should be derived from carbohydrate as a combination of starchy foods and sugary foods.
- Fat soluble vitamin deficiency is common and all pancreatic insufficient patients should be given daily supplements (see Box 11.1).
- Because of the risk of salt depletion, a supplement is recommended for children under 1 year and for those older than 1 in the summer months.
- Dietary supplements are frequently used as a source of additional energy; these include fortified milk shakes, fortified fruit juices and glucose polymers.
- Long-term tube feeding is often instituted when there has been cessation of weight gain over 6 months, or there is evidence of wasting (weight for height ≤80% expected).

> **Box 11.1**   Daily supplements for pancreatic insufficient paediatric patients
>
> - Vitamin A: 8000–10 000 IU (2400–3000 µg).
> - Vitamin D: Ergocalciferal 800 IU (20 µg).
> - Vitamin E:
>   - 50 mg – infants
>   - 100 mg – children aged 1–10 years
>   - 200 mg – above 10 years.
> - Vitamin K: Menandiol 5–10 mg, in liver disease.

Further reading

- Green MR (2001) Nutritional support in cystic fibrosis. In: V Preedy, G Grimble and R Watson (eds) *Nutrition in the Infant*. Greenwich Medical Media, London.
- Patchell C and Johnson T (2000) Feeding children on special diets. In: C Holden and A MacDonald (eds) *Nutrition in Child Health*. Baillière Tindall, Edinburgh.

Neonatal surgery

- Since the first case report of successful long-term PN in an infant with ileal atresia in 1968, this intervention has transformed the prognosis for the surgical newborn patient.
- The majority have congenital anomalies that initially preclude enteral nutrition until recovery from surgery: these include oesophageal, duodenal, ileal or colonic atresia, and abdominal wall defects such as gastroschisis and exomphalos.
- Necrotising enterocolitis (NEC), an acquired condition, is a particular problem in the premature infant and affects around 8% of those weighing less than 1.5 kg; it has a mortality rate of 25–40% and is a cause of considerable morbidity, including short bowel syndrome.
- NEC may also affect term infants with cyanotic heart disease, or following umbilical catheterisation; it is an absolute indication for PN and bowel rest, usually for 10–14 days.
- Gastroschisis is becoming more common for reasons that remain unclear; many of these children have gut dysmotility and some will take weeks or months to tolerate full enteral feeding; the combination of gastroschisis and small bowel atresia is a particularly difficult one since dysmotility and lack of absorptive area combine to preclude full enteral nutrition and increase the risk of cholestasis and liver disease.
- Details of nutritional requirements for infants undergoing surgery are not included here, and advice from an experienced dietitian and pharmacist will be required.
- Management of nutritional support in the long term, i.e. at home, is beyond the scope of this book.

Further reading

- Puntis JWL (2001) Paediatric parenteral nutrition. In: J Payne-James, G Grimble and D Silk (eds) *Artificial Nutrition Support in Clinical Practice* (2e). Greenwich Medical Media, London, pp. 461–84.

Gastrointestinal disorders
Cow's milk protein intolerance

- Milk is the most common food causing intolerance and allergy in young children, affecting around 2.5% of UK infants.
- Cow's milk protein intolerance is the clinical syndrome(s) resulting from sensitisation to one or more proteins in cow's milk.
- Frequently, it resolves spontaneously over the second year of life.
- In most affected children gastrointestinal symptoms (vomiting, diarrhoea, rectal bleeding, colic, constipation) develop in the first 6 months of life.
- Other presentations include: respiratory (wheeze, rhinitis); dermatological (atopic dermatitis, urticaria, laryngeal oedema); behavioural (irritability, crying, milk refusal).
- Diagnosis is based on clinical history, with definite disappearance of symptoms after two dietary eliminations of cow's milk, and recurrence of identical symptoms after one challenge (lactose intolerance and coincidental infection having been excluded).
- Management involves strict avoidance of all forms of cow's milk and dairy products.
- Advice from a paediatric dietitian is required and care must be taken to provide an adequate calcium intake.
- A hydrolysed protein formula feed or soya formula may be given as a milk substitute (around 30% of children will be intolerant of soya protein; occasionally intolerance of peptides in a hydrolysed formula also occurs). These formulas are nutritionally complete for infants. Alternative milks are available for the older child but these frequently have low levels of energy, calcium and vitamins which often need supplementation.

Toddler diarrhoea

- Toddler diarrhoea affects the 6 month–2 years age group and involves frequent passage of loose, offensive stools, often containing undigested food matter (e.g. peas, carrots) in a child who is otherwise well and thriving.
- The underlying mechanism appears to be a rapid gut transit time (ingestion to nappy time for carrot is a good measure!).
- High fibre diets and frequent/excessive consumption of juice exacerbate the problem; increasing dietary fat intake can help (Calogen, a long chain triglyceride supplement can be prescribed, 10 ml tds); trial of a milk free diet can also help some children.

Box 11.2   Oral nutritional requirements to help treat constipation

Encourage intake of the following.

- High fibre breakfast cereal.
- Wholemeal or granary bread.
- Jacket potato with skin.
- Wholemeal pasta and brown rice.
- Wholemeal flour pastry.
- High fibre biscuits/crackers.
- Five servings a day of fruit and vegetables, beans, lentils and other pulses.

Constipation

- Idiopathic constipation is common in the first few years of life.
- Dietary factors include low fluid intake, excessive cow's milk consumption in the toddler (>1 pint/day), and low dietary fibre (non-starch-polysaccharides) intake.
- Cow's milk protein intolerance may be an underlying cause and strict cow's milk exclusion should be tried in children refractory to standard treatment (i.e. laxatives, dietary manipulation and behaviour modification techniques).
- Encourage intake of certain foods (*see* Box 11.2).

Coeliac disease

- Coeliac disease is a condition affecting the small intestine characterised by abnormal mucosa and associated with a lifelong intolerance to gluten; removal of gluten from the diet results in full clinical and histological remission.
- The UK prevalence of coeliac disease in children is around 1 in 2000 to 1 in 6000. Incidence varies according to region.
- Presentation is classically with diarrhoea and failure to thrive, but children may be asymptomatic, or have a range of problems including vomiting, constipation, arthralgia, refractory iron deficiency.
- Diagnosis is often suggested by finding positive anti-endomysial antibodies in the blood, and confirmed by demonstrating the typical histological abnormality (crypt hyperplasia and villus atrophy) in jejunal mucosa, and clinical response to dietary exclusion of gluten.
- In children presenting under 2 years of age, infection or other dietary protein intolerances cause diagnostic confusion; a later gluten challenge is recommended for this age group.
- Treatment is strict dietary gluten avoidance for life; gluten is found in wheat, oats, barley, rye and foods made from these cereals. It is essential that children receive nutritional advice from a dietitian to ensure the diet remains nutritionally adequate. Calcium and vitamin D supplementation may be necessary.
- Many different gluten free dietary products are available to make the diet more varied and easy to follow; detailed information can be provided by dietitians and in publications from the Coeliac Society.
- It is important to make sure that appropriate gluten free meals are provided at school.

- Non-compliance in children results in growth failure and increases the risk of small bowel lymphoma and osteoporosis.

Inflammatory bowel disease

- Growth failure is common in children with inflammatory bowel disease and is seen in 15–40% of patients with Crohn's disease (CD).
- Macronutrient and micronutrient deficiencies frequently occur, particularly in CD.
- Anorexia, abdominal pain, nausea and fear of diarrhoea may restrict dietary intake; mucosal inflammation or gut resection lead to maldigestion, malabsorption and protein losing enteropathy.
- Randomised trials have shown PN to be no better than an elemental or polymeric exclusion diet in inducing remission in CD.
- PN has an important role in peri-operative management of CD patients when enteral nutritional support is not feasible.
- Enteral nutrition is effective as primary therapy in CD but not ulcerative colitis (UC); a 6–8 week exclusion diet consisting only of an elemental or polymeric formula feed is comparable with steroid treatment in inducing remission or treating relapse.
- Polymeric feeds, such as Modulen IBD or conventional paediatric/adult sip feeds, are more palatable than elemental diets, such as Elemental 028 Extra, and children are more likely to take them by mouth.
- CD at any site can respond to an exclusion diet but children with colitis tend to relapse more quickly.
- The mechanisms through which an exclusion diet modulates disease are uncertain; the low fat content of some feeds may mean that pro-inflammatory eicosenoid production from precursor polyunsaturated fatty acids is reduced.
- n-3 marine oils may have a role in attenuating the inflammatory response, being converted into less potent eicosenoids; other feed components including glutamine, fibre and antioxidants are possibly also important in modulating inflammation.
- There is some evidence to suggest that long-term nutritional support (e.g. supplementary night time tube feeds) may help maintain periods of remission in CD.
- Nutritional problems are much less common in UC; if growth failure does occur, nutritional support can usually be given as a high energy/protein diet and sip feeds since the small intestine is unaffected.

Short bowel syndrome

- *See* adult section, p. 109 for further details.
- The term newborn infant has a small intestine approximately 280 cm long; loss of over 50% is likely to have important nutritional consequences and >75% to require long-term PN.
- The ultimate prognosis for survival is good (>90% survival), and the duration of PN relates both to bowel anatomy and quality (e.g. motility).
- Children with as little as 20 cm of small bowel can ultimately become free of PN; the process of adaptation leading to increased absorptive surface area takes place over a long period (years) and includes growth in bowel length and circumference.

- Full enteral feeding is more quickly established in children who retain the colon and ileo–caecal valve.
- Enteral nutrition is initially given at just 1 ml/hr with breast milk if available, or a hydrolysed protein lactose free medium chain triglyceride (MCT) containing feed (e.g. Pregestimil [Mead Johnson], Pepti Junior [Cow & Gate]); milk is increased as tolerated over weeks or months.
- Continuous feeds are better absorbed, but may be more likely to be associated with cholestasis; continuous feeds overnight and bolus feeds in the day are one option with poor feed tolerance or vomiting.
- Hypergastrinaemia may contribute to diarrhoea in the first few months and can be treated with H_2-blockers.
- Cholestyramine 0.1 g/kg qds may help control diarrhoea induced by bile salt malabsorption in the child with a colon; it may interfere with absorption of fat soluble vitamins.
- Sodium depletion as a consequence of stoma losses can be a growth limiting factor even in some children with normal plasma sodium concentration; supplements should be routinely given and urine electrolyte concentration monitored (Na usually kept > 20 mmol/l).
- Attention to oral and psycho-social stimulation, use of pacifiers, tastes of milk (ask for the advice of a speech therapist) are essential if the risk of oral hypersensitivity and later behavioural feeding problems are to be minimised.
- Enteral challenge and progressive diet normalisation takes place over a period of years and depends on each child and residual gastrointestinal tract remaining.
- Long-term complications include gall stones, renal oxalate stones (therefore avoid oxalate containing food sources), vitamin deficiencies, and peri-anastomotic ulceration leading to anaemia.
- Continuing follow up is advisable.

Further reading

- Griffiths AM, Ohisson A, Sherman PM *et al.* (1995) Meta-analysis of enteral nutrition as a primary treatment of active Crohn's disease. *Gastroenterology.* **108**: 1056–67.
- Macdonald S (2001) The gastrointestinal tract. In: V Shaw and M Lawson (eds) *Clinical Paediatric Dietetics* (2e). Blackwell Science, Oxford.
- Patchell C and Johnson T (2000) Feeding children on special diets. In: C Holden and A MacDonald (eds) *Nutrition in Child Health.* Baillière Tindall, Edinburgh.
- Sukhotnik I, Siplovich L, Shiloni E *et al.* (2002) Intestinal adaptation in short-bowel syndrome in infants and children: a collective review. *Pediatr Surg Int.* **18**: 258–63.
- Vanderhoof JA (1996) Short bowel syndrome. *Clinics Perinatol.* **23**: 377–86.
- Wilschanski M, Sherman P, Pencharz P *et al.* (1996) Supplementary enteral nutrition maintains remission paediatric Crohn's disease. *Gut.* **38**: 543–8.

Liver disease

- Protein–energy malnutrition affects over 60% of children with severe liver disease and adversely effects the outcome of liver transplantation.

- Anorexia and fat maldigestion are important contributory causes, particularly in the child with cholestasis.
- Liver disease is associated with fluid retention so that weight measurements as a guide to nutritional status are misleading; mid arm circumference and triceps skinfold thickness below the 10th centile are indicators of the need for nutritional intervention.

Nutritional support in chronic liver disease

- Depending on the severity of disease, energy intake may have to be increased to 140–200% of the estimated average requirement to sustain growth. An experienced dietitian should advise.
- This large increase in energy need is due to an increase in resting energy requirement and, in some cases, fat malabsorption due to a reduction or loss of bile salt production and bile flow.
- Modifications in the type and amount of fat required in the diet are variable; MCTs are often given since their absorption is bile salt independent.
- Energy intake can also be increased through adding glucose polymer to feeds. However, polymer and MCTs increase feed osmolality with the risk of provoking diarrhoea (build up strength of feed slowly to avoid this).
- Protein requirement may also be increased; intake can go up to 4 g/kg/day without provoking hepatic encephalopathy.
- The risks of essential fatty acid and fat soluble vitamin deficiencies are increased; the precise requirements for essential fatty acids are unknown, but large doses of fat soluble vitamins are likely to be necessary (e.g. 5000–20 000 units of vitamin A, 100–800 mg vitamin E, alphacalcidol 20 nanogram/kg [up to 20 kg] and 250–500 nanogram [> 20 kg], and 5–10 mg vitamin K, daily).
- Anorexia experienced by most children with severe liver disease means that tube feeding is often essential if nutritional goals are to be met; an NG tube is used in preference to a gastrostomy because of potential complications related to ascites, variceal formation at the stoma site and the future need for intra-abdominal access during liver transplantation.

Further reading

- France S (2001) The liver and pancreas. In: V Shaw and M Lawson (eds) *Clinical Paediatric Dietetics* (2e). Blackwell Science, Oxford.
- Protheroe SM and Kelly DA (2001) Nutritional requirements and support in liver disease. In: V Preedy, G Grimble and R Watson (eds) *Nutrition in the Infant*. Greenwich Medical Media, London.

Renal disease

Special diets are important in the management of children with impaired renal function, bearing in mind the kidneys' role in excretion of waste products, regulation of water and electrolytes, and metabolic control (e.g. production of 1,25-dihydroxycholecalciferol).

Acute renal failure

- Sudden deterioration in renal function most often occurs in children as a consequence of haemolytic uraemic syndrome.
- Management may be conservative, but short-term dialysis is often required.
- There is not usually a need for specific nutritional intervention.

Nephrotic syndrome

- Most children have minimal change nephrotic syndrome; if repeated courses of steroid treatment are necessary, obesity and linear growth failure may complicate progress.
- Nutritional management involves a balanced diet with adequate protein and energy intake, no added salt, fluid restriction in the initial oedematous phase, and calorie restriction in the child with steroid dependency who is becoming overweight.

Nutritional support in chronic renal failure

- Children with chronic renal failure often have a poor appetite; anorexia increases as plasma urea rises and vomiting may also become a problem.
- The aims of nutritional intervention are to:
  - maintain normal growth
  - regulate protein intake according to growth needs and type of treatment
  - maintain fluid and electrolyte balance
  - regulate calcium and phosphate intake to promote normal bone growth
  - provide an adequate intake of all vitamins and minerals.
- Provision of an adequate energy intake promotes growth and prevents protein catabolism; energy supplements such as glucose polymer, or glucose polymer with fat, and tube feeding may be required.
- Protein restriction is necessary to control uraemia when glomerular filtration rate falls below $50\,\mathrm{ml/min/m^2}$; aim to keep plasma urea concentration $<20\,\mathrm{mmol/l}$.
- If appetite remains good, children are given daily protein allowances; formula fed infants or children receiving tube feeds may require specially modified products.
- Maintenance of normal plasma phosphate and calcium is important if normal bone growth is to occur and rickets and hyperparathyroidism avoided.
- Impaired phosphate excretion requires that dietary phosphate intake is limited; a low phosphate formula may be required for infants and in older children dairy produce and phosphate rich foods should be restricted.
- If dietary restriction fails to control plasma phosphate, calcium carbonate containing phosphate binding tablets can be taken with meals and snacks.
- Potassium restriction becomes necessary when children are approaching end-stage renal failure; high potassium foods must be avoided (e.g. bananas, potato, fruit cake, chocolate, biscuits, fruit juice, crisps, milk).
- In end-stage renal failure a low salt diet may also be advised, particularly if blood pressure is raised or fluid intake restricted.

- A multivitamin supplement is often needed to ensure that children meet their recommended nutrient intake; in addition, vitamin D supplements, such as alphacalcidol, are necessary to replace 1,25-dihydroxycholecalciferol normally produced by the kidneys.

Further reading

- Coleman J (2001) The kidney. In: V Shaw and M Lawson (eds) *Clinical Paediatric Dietetics* (2e) Blackwell Science, Oxford, pp. 158–81.

Haematology/oncology

- Leukaemia accounts for 30–45% of childhood cancers, lymphomas 9–15%, and solid tumours (e.g. medulloblastoma, Wilm's, neuroblastoma, etc) for around 40%.
- Malnutrition and cachexia are frequent consequences of childhood malignancies.
- The prevalence of malnutrition ranges from 6–50% depending on the type, stage and location of the tumour.
- Weight measurement is inaccurate as an indicator of nutritional status in children with a large tumour mass, and mid upper arm circumference (MUAC) and skinfold thickness measurements are more reliable methods of assessing nutritional status.
- Rather than conserving energy and protein reserves in response to starvation, the patient with malignant disease may increase energy expenditure, proteolysis and gluconeogenesis, more characteristic of acute metabolic stress.
- Alterations in carbohydrate metabolism include decreased glucose tolerance and increased lactate production; both protein synthesis and degradation are increased, as are lipolysis and fatty acid oxidation.
- Malignant cachexia appears to be mainly related to the increased metabolic demands of the tumour burden; cytokines such as tumour necrosis factor (TNF) may play an important role.
- Side-effects of treatment that impact on nutritional status include infection, diarrhoea, nausea and vomiting, stomatitis, renal damage, and altered taste perception.
- Learned food aversion associated with nausea inducing treatment is a well recognised phenomenon and may lead to anticipatory vomiting.
- *See* Box 11.3 for pointers to likely need for nutritional intervention.

Box 11.3 Pointers to likely need for nutritional intervention in haematology/oncology

- Loss >5% body weight.
- Weight for height <90%.
- Drop of weight across two centile lines.
- Food intake <70% of estimated requirement.
- Bone marrow transplant patient.

Nutritional support

- The aims of nutritional support are to reverse the malnutrition seen at diagnosis, to prevent a deterioration in nutritional status during treatment and to promote normal growth.
- Nutritional support should be considered a major part of therapy; there is no evidence that extra nutrients supplied promote tumour growth (i.e. feed the tumour).
- Children at low nutritional risk require high energy supplements that can be taken by mouth; they benefit from flexibility in meal times and menus, i.e. letting them eat what they want when they want (not always easy in a hospital setting).
- In children with an inadequate oral energy intake enteral tube feeding should be used; this is usually well tolerated and improves wellbeing, even in children undergoing intensive chemotherapy.
- Usually a whole protein feed will be tolerated; if not, a protein hydrolysate may be substituted.
- PN is reserved for those children with severe gastrointestinal symptoms relating to underlying disease, chemotherapy or radiotherapy.

Bone marrow transplantation

- Priming chemotherapy often causes severe nausea, vomiting and oral ulceration and in bone marrow transplant patients is associated with diarrhoea and protein losing enteropathy.
- PN may be required, and enteral feeds should be prepared in a manner that renders them low in bacterial load ('clean feeds'), given that patients are immunosuppressed.

Further reading

- Papadopoulou A (1998) Nutritional support in children undergoing bone marrow transplant. *Clin Nutr.* **17**: 57–63.
- Smith DE (1992) An investigation of supplementary nasogastric feeding in malnourished children undergoing treatment for malignancy: results of pilot study. *J Hum Nutr Diet.* **5**: 85–91.
- Ward E (2001) Childhood cancers. In: V Shaw and M Lawson (eds) *Clinical Paediatric Dietetics* (2e). Blackwell Science, Oxford.

Neurodisability
Feeding problems

- Around 15–20 000 children in the UK suffer from cerebral palsy, of whom 40–50% have feeding difficulties that have implications for nutritional status.
- 85% of children with spastic quadriplegia have severe feeding problems.
- These are often related to difficulty getting food into the mouth, impaired chewing and swallowing mechanisms, and vomiting.

- Vomiting is frequently due to underlying gastro-oesophageal reflux disease.
- Children may be anorexic, have aversive behaviour to feeding, cannot request or obtain food, may not be able to wield eating utensils, and have inadequate assistance or supervision.
- Among other consequences, malnutrition may lead to impairment of growth and development, immunodeficiency, apathy and depression.

Assessment of feeding problems

- Should be multidisciplinary, e.g. caregiver, paediatrician, dietitian, speech and language therapist (SALT), occupational therapist, and physiotherapist.
- A careful feeding history is essential together with an assessment of oromotor function, nutritional status, neurological deficit, respiratory, physical ability and psychological state.
- Weight, MUAC, triceps or subscapular skinfold thickness and limb/spinal length may be easier to measure than length in children with scoliosis or spasticity.
- Issues to be considered include the safety, nutritional adequacy, enjoyment and duration of meal times.
- A videofluoroscopy is a specialised investigation to look at swallowing mechanism and determine the risk of aspiration during oral feeding and this is usually supervised by a SALT.
- Feed thickeners may be necessary in those with a degree of dysphagia.
- Children who cannot maintain an adequate oral intake of food or fluids will need supplementary tube feeding.
- Long-term tube feeding is better done *via* a gastrostomy than NG tube; a gastrostomy is more acceptable cosmetically, less likely to become displaced, and improves the quality of life for carers and child.
- If a trial of NG feeding does not unmask or provoke significant gastro-oesophageal reflux, a gastrostomy can be placed without concomitant antireflux surgery.

Nutritional management

- Estimating energy requirement is problematic; limited activity decreases energy expenditure whereas spasticity, athetosis, convulsions and infection increase energy need.
- In general energy requirements are less than those for non-disabled children (*see* Table 9.3).
- Protein should provide at least 10% of total energy intake.
- Mineral, trace element, iron and vitamin supplements may be required due to the low energy load of diet.
- Increased nutritional intake by mouth can be achieved through simple measures such as change of seating and posture, and feeding food appropriate to the developmental age of the child.
- Desensitisation programmes are effective in children with aversive behaviour and pureed or thickened feeds can help overcome swallowing difficulties.
- Gastrostomy is necessary for long-term feeding in children who cannot maintain an adequate oral intake or who have unsafe airway and are at risk of aspiration.

- Following institution of tube feeding, weight gain should be carefully monitored; children with cerebral palsy increase their fat stores more easily than lean tissue mass and excessive weight gain should be avoided.

Further reading

- Allott L (2000) Feeding children with special needs. In: C Holden and A MacDonald (eds) *Nutrition and Child Health*. Baillière Tindall, London.
- Stevenson RD and Meyers R (2001) Nutrition in the child with disabilities. In: V Preedy, G Grimble and R Watson (eds) *Nutrition in the Infant*. Greenwich Medical Media, London.
- Sullivan PB and Rosenbloom L (eds) (1996) *Feeding the Disabled Child. Clinics in Developmental Medicine No 140*. MacKeith Press, Cambridge.

The premature newborn
Parenteral nutritional support

- Low nutritional reserve and high energy requirements indicate that nutritional support should be instituted early in these sick and vulnerable infants ($< 1500\,g$ birthweight).
- Undernutrition is thought to adversely effect later neurodevelopmental outcome.
- PN is used more widely in the premature newborn than any other group of paediatric patients.
- The principle indication for PN is immaturity of gastrointestinal function since gastric stasis, abdominal distension and infrequent stooling mean enteral nutrition must be cautiously advanced until gut motor development has matured.
- There is an additional concern that too rapid incrementation of milk feeds will greatly increase the risk of NEC, a serious complication of prematurity with high mortality and morbidity.
- The most appropriate feeding strategy for prevention of NEC is uncertain, but breast milk is probably protective, as is slow build up to full milk feeding over the first 10 days of life.
- Significant risks of PN include glucose intolerance (with osmotic diuresis), hypertriglyceridaemia, central venous catheter sepsis and cholestasis.
- Variable fluid and electrolyte requirements mean that individualised PN prescriptions are often desirable, although there is also scope for use of standard feeds.
- There is considerable variation in the practice of nutritional support in different neonatal units reflecting lack of an evidence base. However, there has been a general move towards more early and aggressive intervention.
- Aim to begin PN within the first 24 hours if possible; also begin minimal enteral feeding (use mother's or bank breast milk if available) – 1 ml/kg/hr. Typically 0.5 ml every 2 hours is given for babies less than 30 weeks' gestation and 1 ml every 2 hours for babies over 30 weeks' gestation.
- Subsequently build up parenteral nutrient intake over several days; for nutritional requirements *see* Table 11.1.

Table 11.1   Estimated nutrient intake needed to achieve fetal weight gain. (From Ziegler *et al.*, 2002)

Body weight (g)	500–700	700–900	900–1200	1200–1500	1500–1800
Fetal weight					
Gain g/day	13	16	20	24	26
g/kg/day	21	20	19	18	16
Protein (g)					
Urinary/skin loss	1.0	1.0	1.0	1.0	1.0
Growth (accretion)[a]	2.5	2.5	2.5	2.4	2.2
Required intake: parenteral	3.5	3.5	3.5	3.4	3.2
Required intake: enteral[b]	4.0	4.0	4.0	3.9	3.6
Energy (kcal)					
Loss	60	60	60	60	60
Resting expenditure	45	45	50	50	50
Misc. expenditure	15	15	15	20	20
Growth (accretion)[c]	29	32	36	38	39
Required intake: parenteral	89	92	101	108	109
Required intake: enteral[d]	105	108	119	127	128
Protein/energy (g/100 kcal)					
Parenteral	3.9	4.1	3.5	3.1	2.9
Enteral	3.8	3.7	3.4	3.1	2.8

[a] Includes correction for 90% efficiency of conversion from dietary to body protein.
[b] Same as parenteral but assuming 88% absorption of dietary protein.
[c] Energy accretion plus 10 kcal/kg/day cost of growth.
[d] Assuming 85% absorption of dietary energy.

Enteral feeding

- Respiratory disease or immaturity of suck and swallow mechanisms mean that most premature infants (<37 weeks' gestation) will be fed *via* an NG tube.
- Orogastric tubes are favoured for infants with respiratory distress by some units.
- When fully established, daily milk volumes are in the order of 150–180 ml/kg.
- There is ongoing debate regarding use of continuous or bolus NG feeds until full volumes are established.
- Continuous feeds may be better tolerated in infants with immature gut motor function, and are associated with a lower energy expenditure and possible improved weight gain.
- Bolus feeds are thought by some to be more 'physiological' and may be better at stimulating gut hormone release, promoting motor development and bile flow.

- Mother's milk appears to be protective against NEC and tolerated better than formula feed in sick infants; it may be expressed milk from the baby's own mother (maternal EBM) or donor milk, expressed by feeding mothers in the community and given to a milk bank.
- Milk banking became less popular in the late 1980s due to concerns regarding nutritional adequacy of donor milk (low energy and mineral content) and the potential for viral transmission; there has been a recent resurgence of interest partly due to the fact that milk fortifiers can now be used where necessary to make good the nutritional deficiencies whilst hopefully preserving the beneficial effects of breast milk. Breast milk fortifiers available are: Nutriprem Breast Milk Fortifier (Cow & Gate), Eoprotin (Milupa), Enfamil (Mead Johnson), SMA Breast Milk Fortifier (SMA).
- When EBM is not available a preterm formula milk is used with higher energy density, protein and mineral content more suited to the needs of the preterm infant than a standard infant formula. The preterm formulas are: Nutriprem 1 (Cow & Gate), Osterprem (Farleys), SMA Low Birthweight (SMA), Prematil (Milupa).
- Infants are often discharged from the neonatal unit around the time they would have been born if premature delivery had not occurred; they often weigh much less than an average term infant and their nutritional requirements for catch up growth are now being taken into account through provision of nutrient enriched post-discharge formulas such as Nutriprem 2 (Cow & Gate) and Premcare (Farleys).

Further reading

- ASPEN Board of Directors and Clinical Guidelines Task Force (2002) Guidelines for the Use of Parenteral and Enteral Nutrition in Adults and Paediatric Patients. *JPEN.* **26** (Suppl 1): 1SA–138SA.
- Cooke RJ and Embleton ND (2000) Feeding issues in preterm infants. *Arch Dis Child Fetal Neonatal Ed.* **83**: F215–18.
- Klein CJ (2002) Nutrient requirements for preterm infant formulas. A report from the American Society for Nutritional Science, Life Sciences Research Ofice. *J Nutr.* **132** (Suppl 1): 1395S–1578S.
- Ziegler EE, Thureen PJ and Carlson SJ (2002) Aggressive nutrition in the very low birthweight infant. *Clin Perinatol.* **29**: 225–44.

Critical illness

Many of the physiological and clinical principles that govern the nutritional care of the critically ill child are similar to those in adult medicine. Chapter 7, nutritional support in the critically ill patient (p. 92), should therefore be referred to, although it should be noted that the critically ill child's protein and energy requirements will differ from those of adults.

Nutritional management

- The aim of nutritional support for children on intensive care is to minimise negative energy and protein balance, maintain tissue function, and maintain gut function.

- Route of feeding tends to be NG due to endotracheal intubation as this is the easiest route of administration.
- There are no specific recommendations for energy and protein for the critically ill child. Energy and protein needs are derived from dietary reference values and are considered alongside clinical and biochemical parameters.
- Early enteral feeding reduces complications and initiation of enteral feeds within 24 hours is a standard for most units.
- Paralysis and sedation will reduce gut motility and gastric aspirates can be high. Prokinetics such as domperidone are useful if this is a problem. Standard age appropriate enteral feeds are usually well tolerated.
- Trans-pyloric feeding is an option if gastric stasis is an issue. Drug–nutrient interactions are an important consideration. Liaison with the unit pharmacist is critical.
- PN should only be considered when the gut is not functioning.
- There is no evidence for the use of novel substrates in the critically ill paediatric population.

Further reading

- Fung EB (2000) Estimating energy expenditure in critically ill adults and children. *AACN Clin Issues*. **11**: 480–97.
- Irving SY, Simone SD, Hicks FW *et al.* (2000) Nutrition for the critically ill child: enteral and parenteral support. *AACN Clin Issues*. **11**: 541–58.
- Iyer PU (2002) Nutritional support in the critically ill child. *Indian J Pediatr*. **69**: 405–10.

PART 4

Ethics of nutritional support

CHAPTER 12

Ethics of nutritional support

Introduction

Ethical principles of nutritional support are a difficult area that many professionals prefer to avoid. However, if best practice is to be achieved, then avoidance of the issue is not an option.

Ethics is a complex science and there are many different approaches to it. Detailed discussion is beyond the scope of this book, and the interested reader should refer to the further reading list below.

This chapter is designed to be a pragmatic guide for the practising healthcare professional. One approach favoured by many clinicians experienced in nutritional support is the 'four principles' approach of autonomy, non-maleficence, beneficence and justice (*see* Table 12.1). While it can be argued that this is a simplistic overview of a very complex area, it is a very helpful one to guide practice in nutritional support.

Ethical principles applied to nutrition

- The provision of food and water constitutes 'basic care' and is mandatory for all patients.
- The administration of nutrition *via* feeding tubes is a medical intervention and requires consent.
- Some patients may wish to eat but cannot, e.g. difficulty in chewing, poor appetite, apathy/depression, weakness. Therefore food needs to be presented in an appetising and appropriate way with encouragement and assistance offered where necessary.

Table 12.1   The four principles

Autonomy	The principle of self-determination, i.e. it recognises patients' rights and lets them decide their own destiny
Non-maleficence	The deliberate avoidance of harm (to the patient)
Beneficence	The provision of benefit
Justice	The fair and equitable provision of available medical resources for all

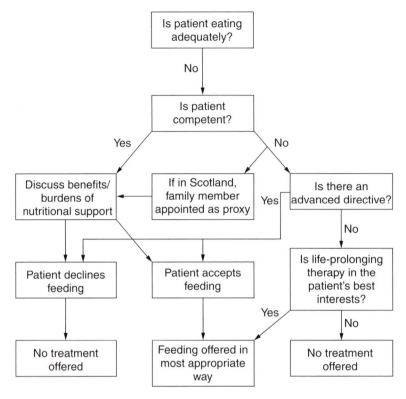

Figure 12.1 Decision-making algorithm for nutritional support.

- People at the end of their lives may eat little. This is a natural phenomenon and should be accepted.
- If, despite encouragement ± use of oral nutritional supplements, a patient's oral intake is still insufficient, consideration needs to be given to artificial nutritional support, which in the main implies tube feeding.
- When determining whether tube feeding may be appropriate, consider the following.
  - Is any reversibility likely in the underlying illness that may indicate more aggressive intervention would be appropriate?
  - What quality of life is going to be preserved/regained?
  - Is nutritional support just going to prolong the dying period for patients with poor prognosis?
- *See* Figure 12.1.

Competence

After consideration of whether nutritional support is appropriate, the next step is to determine whether the patient is competent to consent. *See* Box 12.1 for the definition of competence.

Box 12.1 Definition of competence

- Ability to understand what the medical treatment is, its purpose and why it is being proposed.
- Ability to understand benefits, risks and alternatives.
- Ability to understand consequences of refusal.
- Ability to retain information for long enough to make an effective decision.

The 'competent' patient

- The situation should be presented to the patient in a clear and unbiased way.
- Decisions should be free from pressure.
- Communication of the decision should be interpretable, but not necessarily verbal, e.g. hand squeeze.
- The patient's decision is binding, however irrational that may appear, and even if that decision may result in their dying.
- A clinician has no obligation to treat/intervene against his/her judgement, providing that this is in accordance with a widely held professional view. Should a situation arise where pressure is being put on by patient or family for feeding to be instituted, the clinician can either offer to seek a second opinion and/or to get advice from hospital solicitors or defence organisations.

The 'incompetent' patient

- If the patient is not competent, as per the stipulations in Box 12.1, the following need to be considered.
  - In Scotland a family member can act as proxy and have the same legal rights as the patient would have done. Therefore, in this situation, the matter can be considered as per a 'competent' patient.
  - In England, Wales and most European countries family and carers can express opinions, but these are not legally binding.
  - Is there an advanced directive (AD)? (*See* Box 12.2.)
- Where there is no AD and the situation is not in Scotland, the treating clinician has the responsibility of making a decision in the patient's 'best interest', taking into account the ethical principles set out in Table 12.1.
- Although family/carer views have no legal standing (except in Scotland), they should be taken into account.
- There should be wide discussion with all relevant professionals – nurses, other allied professions, general practitioners and relevant community-based staff.
- The concept of 'quality of life' is vague and means different things to different people. Withholding nutritional support on the basis of 'no quality of life' needs careful discussion with all concerned, and taking into account the underlying disease process.

Box 12.2 Advance directives

- ADs are recognised in UK law (although they have not been adequately tested in the Courts).
- If there is an AD then this needs to be adhered to, whether written or oral.
- Written ADs will usually have been drawn up by a patient ± family and sometimes with the help of a solicitor, but usually without any input from a healthcare professional. Most will be worded in a very vague 'generic' way, e.g. 'no artificial feeding if I am rendered incapable'. This can make it difficult for clinicians subsequently to interpret when a specific clinical situation presents itself. For example, if a patient comes in unconscious from a stroke with the above AD, is the clinician bound to it absolutely even when there is a chance of recovery over the following few weeks? If the clinician does follow the AD, he/she will be depriving the patient of necessary support during the crucial early weeks; if the clinician does not, he/she risks legal action.
- Verbal ADs can be even more tenuous and difficult to interpret, and often have to be taken 'on trust' by the clinical team when they are relayed (usually) by a family member.
- If there is doubt, hospital solicitors should be involved.

- If there is uncertainty, a second opinion from a senior clinician is appropriate.
- If doubt still remains, hospital solicitors and/or defence organisations should be involved.

Withholding and withdrawing nutritional support

- There is no difference in legal or ethical terms between the two, although emotionally it can be more difficult to withdraw.
- While a deliberate act to kill a patient is unlawful, omission of a treatment that may allow death to occur as a consequence of the disease process is *not* unlawful.
- Tube feeding should be withheld if it is futile, e.g. advanced cancer, end-stage dementia, *but* each case needs to be considered on its own merits.
- There can often be a case for a time-limited trial of therapy, e.g. a trial of NG feeding for several weeks after a stroke, but withdrawal after a pre-determined length of time (e.g. 4 weeks) if there have been no signs of recovery.
- Where nutritional support is to be withheld or withdrawn it is generally advisable to seek a second opinion. Some clinicians may also feel more comfortable contacting their defence organisation and/or hospital solicitors.
- Currently in the UK the only situation in adult practice that requires a Court order to withdraw feeding is the persistent vegetative state (PVS).
- If nutritional support is to be withheld/withdrawn, food and water with assistance if appropriate should still be offered, as per 'basic care'. Artificial hydration (IV or SC), however, should not be started/continued, as this will prolong the dying process and certainly would not be in the patient's best interests.

Nutritional support in specific situations
Dementia

- There is general agreement, supported in the literature, that artificial nutritional support in end-stage dementia is inappropriate. How 'end-stage' is defined, however, is unclear.
- It should be remembered that oral intake does diminish as the disease progresses. This is a natural phenomenon and should be accepted.
- Tube feeding in these patients should be the exception rather than the rule.

Anorexia nervosa

- As a clinician, if a patient with anorexia is referred for tube feeding, a very close collaboration with a psychiatrist is essential. The underlying illness is primarily a psychiatric one and there must be an ongoing plan of psychiatric therapy.
- Tube feeding should only be considered if all other options have been explored, and usually only when physical health is threatened.
- Whatever nutritional therapy is undertaken, clear nutritional and anthropometric goals need to be set.
- If the patient is unwilling to accept tube feeding, it can be done under the Mental Health Act. Psychiatric colleagues will need to advise.
- If necessary, restraint methods can be instituted, but great care must be taken not to infringe basic human rights, irrespective of whether the patient is under Section.

Cancer

- Artificial nutritional support in terminal cancer is not carried out in the UK nearly as much as it is in many other European countries or the US, probably because many professionals do not even consider it.
- Where demise is not imminent, and oral intake is poor, then artificial nutritional support should be considered. Sometimes PN may be necessary if there is intestinal failure, e.g. as a result of widespread abdominal disease. The pros and cons need to be discussed carefully with the patient and he/she should be left to decide.

Considerations in paediatric practice

- The same principles for infants and children apply as for adults.
- In paediatric practice there are some situations in which withdrawing or withholding artificial nutritional support can be ethically justified. Examples would be severe brain damage and progressive neurodegenerative disorders.
- A young person under 16 years of age may have the capacity to decide for themselves. If this is the case then they should be allowed to do so.
- Where a child lacks capacity to decide, a person with parental responsibility may authorise or refuse treatment.

- There are guidelines from the Royal College of Paediatrics and Child Health on withdrawing and withholding treatment, although little specific on nutritional support. However, the General Medical Council's advice on nutrition and hydration offers guiding principles and a good practice framework (applicable to adults and children).

Further reading

- Beauchamp T and Childress J (2001) *Principles of Biomedical Ethics* (5e). Oxford University Press, New York, US.
- General Medical Council (2002) *Withholding and Withdrawing Life-prolonging Treatments: good practice in decision-making*. General Medical Council, London.
- Lennard-Jones JE (1999) *Ethical and Legal Aspects of Clinical Hydration and Nutritional Support. A report from the British Association for Parenteral and Enteral Nutrition*. BAPEN, Maidenhead.
- Lennard-Jones JE (1999) Giving or withholding fluid and nutrients: ethical and legal aspects. *J R Coll Physicians Lond*. **33**: 39–45.
- MacFie J (2000) Ethical and legal considerations in the provision of nutritional support to the perioperative patient. *Curr Opin Nutr Metab Care*. **3**: 23–9.
- Royal College of Paediatrics and Child Health (1997) *Withholding or Withdrawing Life Saving Treatment in Children. A framework for practice*. Royal College of Paediatrics and Child Health, London.

Index